THE FAMILY GUIDE TO VITAMINS, HERBS, AND SUPPLEMENTS

THE FAMILY GUIDE TO VITAMINS, HERBS, AND SUPPLEMENTS

Deborah Mitchell

A Lynn Sonberg Book

St. Martin's Paperbacks

Notice: This book is intended as a reference volume only, not as a medical manual. The information given here is designed to help you make informed decisions about your health. It is not intended as a substitute for any treatment that may have been prescribed by your doctor. If you suspect that you have a medical problem, we urge you to seek competent medical help.

Mention of specific companies, organizations, or authorities in this book does not imply endorsement by the author or publisher, nor does mention of specific companies, organizations, or authorities imply that they endorse this book, its author or the publisher.

Internet addresses given in this book were accurate at the time it went to press.

THE FAMILY GUIDE TO VITAMINS, HERBS, AND SUPPLEMENTS

Copyright © 2011 by Lynn Sonberg Book Associates.

Cover photo of alternative remedies by Image Source / Getty Images; photo of peppers by Nathan Blaney / Getty Images.

All rights reserved.

For information address St. Martin's Press, 175 Fifth Avenue, New York, NY 10010.

EAN: 978-0-312-53417-2

Printed in the United States of America

St. Martin's Paperbacks edition / January 2011

St. Martin's Paperbacks are published by St. Martin's Press, 175 Fifth Avenue, New York, NY 10010.

10 9 8 7 6 5 4 3 2 1

CONTENTS

PART II: COMMON AILMENTS THAT CAN AFFECT YOU AND YOUR FAMILY   71

PART III: NATURAL SUPPLEMENTS FOR YOU AND YOUR FAMILY 157

Nutritional Supplements

Herbal Supplements

INTRODUCTION

The majority of adults in America are already doing it, and chances are because you picked up this book, you are doing it too—or are ready to start. Of course we are talking about taking nutritional supplements, which I believe is one of the best ways you can gain control over your health and the health of your family.

In today's uncertain healthcare environment, taking control of your own health and that of your family is one of the most important things you can do. Incorporating preventive medicine steps into your lifestyle is the most logical and economical way to health care, because you don't have to treat what you don't get! When you practice healthful habits, including eating nourishing foods, exercising regularly, and getting enough sleep, you are protecting yourself against illness and disease. Taking nutritional supplements and herbal remedies is another important step you can take to protect yourself and your family against everything from annoying symptoms to life-altering ailments.

Yet choosing the most appropriate supplements and remedies for yourself and your family can be a challenge. When you walk into a pharmacy or natural health store or even a supermarket, the aisles and aisles of nutritional supplements and herbal remedies can take your breath away. How do you know which supplements are best to protect and maintain your family's overall health? Which nutritional supplements and herbal remedies are most effective for certain ailments and symptoms? What are the safest dosages to take? Which supplements and herbal remedies are safe for your children? Are there any risks associated with taking nutritional supplements and herbal remedies?

Because nutritional and herbal supplements are not subject to the same strict regulations imposed by the Food and Drug Administration (FDA) on over-the-counter and prescription drugs, consumers often rely on information provided by the makers of the supplements themselves and whatever else they can gather from other sources. How can you decipher the often confusing and conflicting information about all these products? The search for reliable information can take a lot of time and effort, unless you can find it in a comprehensive, concise source.

You have found that source.

WHY YOU NEED THIS BOOK

In this family guide to nutritional supplements and herbal remedies, providing detailed information on safety is a prime concern. For example, just because nutritional supplements and herbs are "natural" does not mean they are completely safe. If supplements are not taken as recommended, some people may experience side effects. According to the American Association of Poison Control Centers, more than 1.6 million reports of adverse effects related to taking vitamins, minerals, essential oils, herbs, and other supplements were reported to the Centers from 1983 through 2004, including 251,799 that were serious enough to require hospitalization.

We don't tell you this to frighten you, but to let you know that it is important to treat nutritional and herbal supplements with the respect that they deserve. After all, you and your family want to take them because they work, so you know they have power!

And so do you. In this book we explore dozens of the more common ailments and diseases that can affect you and your family and the nutritional and herbal supplements that you can take to prevent or treat these conditions. Equally if not more important, we also discuss what you need to know about common but critical nutritional supplements to boost the immune system and help preserve and maintain your and your family's overall health and well-being.

HOW TO USE THIS BOOK

This book is divided into three parts, each of which contains information that complements each other. In Part 1, "Taking Care of You and Your Family," we discuss topics that will help you make informed decisions when you are ready to turn to Part 2, "Common Ailments," and Part 3, "Natural Supplements," to select supplements for you and your family.

For example, in chapter 1 we explore issues that most concern parents when they are considering giving supplements to their children: does my child need supplements, which supplements are safest and most effective, how do I choose supplements, are herbal remedies safe for my children, and how do I choose herbal supplements for my kids. The answers you get here will help you decide which dietary and herbal supplements may be best for your child's health and well-being and which help prevent or treat certain common ailments.

Chapter 2 is for you and other adults in your life. Just like children are not little adults, adults are not big children; the nutritional needs are different for each. In chapter 2 we discuss some of the nutritional needs of adults as they go through the decades; how those needs change, especially during pregnancy and in the senior years; choosing herbal remedies for adults; the impact of medications on nutrients; and the impact of diet on medication. These latter two issues are of particular concern to older adults, who often are taking multiple drugs. A review of all these topics can help you as you decide which nutritional and herbal supplements covered in the subsequent parts of the book can best suit your needs and those of your loved ones.

Chapter 3 is like an insurance policy, because it provides information that will safeguard your and your family's health against environmental harm from foods, assists you in finding a qualified healthcare provider, helps you understand the terms you will encounter when shopping for the nutritional and herbal supplements we discuss in Part 3, and explains the tools you should have at home for your family's natural medicine survival kit.

Once you are armed with information from the first 3 chapters, you are ready to make informed decisions about which nutritional and/or herbal supplements will best suit your and your family's needs. All of the entries for the ailments discussed in detail in Part 2 include suggested nutritional and herbal supplements that can be used as treatments, with specific dosing information for both children and adults. Once you have chosen one or more supplements that you want to consider or learn more about, you can turn to Part 3, where we provide details on each of the vitamins, minerals, and herbal remedies mentioned in Part 2.

Remember, you should always check with your doctor or healthcare provider before you or your loved ones take a new supplement. It is best to consult a professional who has expertise in natural medicine, such as a naturopath. We offer help on how to find such providers in chapter 3.

PART I

Taking Care of You and Your Family

CHAPTER ONE

Children and Natural Supplements

It's automatic: You're a parent, you have a child, you worry. Even before he or she emerged from the womb, you were concerned about your child's health, and that concern is ongoing. Perhaps you have decided to introduce your child to natural supplements as a way to protect his or her health. Right now, only one-third of children ages two through 17 take nutritional supplements, according to a recent report, but many, many more could benefit from them. And your child can be one of them!

Parents everywhere know—or they find out very quickly—that keeping kids healthy can be a challenge. Kids often are picky eaters, they fall and get bruises and broken bones, they are exposed to germs, and they contract childhood illnesses. As a parent you face many challenges, but there are also many steps you can take to help ensure the health and well-being of your children.

Part of that effort, and one that is growing in popularity, is to give children natural supplements—vitamins, minerals, and other nutrients, as well as herbal remedies—for a wide variety of reasons, ranging from boosting the immune system to fighting an episode of common cold or flu or earache, to making sure they get all the nutrients they need while they go through a picky-eater stage. More and more parents are turning away from antibiotics and other prescription and over-the-counter medications and supporting the health of their children with natural supplements.

This chapter explores why infants, young children, and adolescents need supplements, how to get children to take them, how to choose supplements for children, and which additives to avoid. It also discusses different herbal remedies that are safe for children and how they can be used to prevent and treat certain illnesses and diseases, as well as promote overall health and well-being. Once you gain a better understanding of how your child can benefit from natural supplements, you will be better able to make an informed decision about which supplements to choose when you turn to Parts 2 and 3 for details on natural supplements and the conditions they can treat.

DO YOUR CHILDREN NEED NUTRITIONAL SUPPLEMENTS?

Will all the parents whose children eat the daily recommended number of fruits and vegetables, who get no more than 20 percent of their calories from fat, who get enough calcium for strong bones, and who eat only a limited amount of sugary foods and beverages and other junk foods please stand up and take a bow. Did anyone stand up? If so, you are in the minority.

As a parent, you are also in the minority if you provide nutritional supplements for your children. The latest figures published in the February 2009 issue of the *Archives of Pediatrics and Adolescent Medicine* reported that 34 percent of children and adolescents ages two to 17 use vitamin and mineral supplements, which means 66 percent of them do not. You may be among the majority of parents who do not give your children supplements but you are thinking about it. You may be asking yourself: Do my children need nutritional supplements?

In a perfect world, children might not need to take any nutritional supplements. But in our stressful, fast-paced, fast-food world, they are an asset. Pediatricians often recommend a daily multivitamin or mineral supplement, or even additional individual nutritional supplements, for:

- Picky eaters who do not eat enough food
- Kids who do not eat regular, well-balanced meals consisting mainly of fresh, whole foods
- Kids who have chronic health conditions such as digestive problems or asthma, especially if they are taking medications. (Do not give your child any supplements if he or she is taking medications until you talk to your doctor.)
- Active kids, especially those who are heavily involved with sports
- Kids who eat a lot of fast foods and/or processed foods
- Kids who are on a limited diet such as dairy-free (may need calcium supplements), vegetarian (may need iron), or other restrictions
- Kids who drink a lot of carbonated sodas, which can leach essential nutrients from their bodies

When you look at this list, it seems that it covers just about child you know. And that's okay, because taking supplements is an easy yet effective way to protect your child's health.

Supplements Can Be Good Medicine

The number one reason by a landslide (75 percent) why parents give supplements to their children is to promote overall health and wellness, followed by supplementing their nutrition (22 percent) and to treat colds (5 percent). Interviews with 8,000 consumers show that of parents who buy nutritional products for children younger than 12 years of age, 43 percent buy multiple vitamins and 38 percent buy vitamins that are specifically labeled for use by children. Parents who buy minerals are looking for calcium (45 percent), zinc (22 percent), and fluoride (15 percent). We discuss all of these and many other supplements in this book.

We know that it's difficult to make sure your children eat nutritious food all the time. For some parents, getting their child to eat a vegetable—any vegetable—is a major challenge, and a fight they feel they have lost. The term "picky eater" seems to apply to more and more children. Many children will latch onto a few specific foods and refuse to eat anything else. One mother says her five-year-old will not eat anything except macaroni and cheese, peanut butter and jelly, and grapes, no matter how creative she tries to be. Another says her six-year-old daughter will not eat anything that is green, "squishy," or has leaves. Does this sound familiar?

Even if your child does eat some fruits and vegetables and stays away from most sugary and junk foods, other factors can deplete nutrient levels, just like they can in adults: stress, environmental pollutants, lack of sufficient sleep, and use of medications (including antibiotics). Add to this the fact that children are growing and so need optimal nutrition, essential ingredients they will not get if they eat lots of processed and/or fast food, which offer empty calories and poor nutritional value.

Another important reason children can benefit from supplements is to boost their immune system. Did you know that a child's immune system is not fully developed until he or she is 14 years old? Yet that doesn't stop the bacteria, viruses, fungi, parasites, and other disease-causing organisms from attacking. In fact, they have a much better chance of taking hold and causing symptoms or disease because the child's immune system is not up to speed. That's why eating a healthful diet and taking supplements to boost the immune system can be your child's best defense against illness.

Food Versus Supplements

It is important to remember that supplements are exactly that: they are meant to *supplement* the diet, not replace it. Whole, natural foods are still the best way for your children (and you) to get the nutrients that are essential for health. To help you along, the U.S. Department of Agriculture (USDA) and the Institute of Medicine created a food pyramid just for kids, but many experts believe the USDA should have been stricter when it comes to some of its guidelines for grains (should insist on whole grains), dairy (should insist on low- and non-fat), and sweets (should eliminate them). In the book *Real Food for Healthy Kids,* authors Tracey Seaman and Tanya Wenman Steel have taken the USDA guidelines and expounded on them, providing parents with a solid foundation from which to select foods for their children. Here are some guidelines by age and an explanation of the categories.

RECOMMENDED FOOD INTAKE DAILY FOR CHILDREN AGES 2–17

Food Group	Ages 2–4	Ages 5–11	Ages 12+
Vegetables	1 cup	2 cups	3 cups
Fruits	1 cup	1 1/2 cups	2 cups
Grains	3 oz	5–6 oz	6 oz
Meat & Beans	2–3 oz	5 oz	5–6 oz
Dairy	2 cups	3 cups	3 cups
Oils	3 tsp	4 tsp	5–6 tsp
Fats & Sweets	Limited	Limited	Limited

Vegetables: Best choices are dark, bright veggies, such as spinach, carrots, sweet potatoes, bell peppers, and tomatoes. Starchy veggies such as corn and baking potatoes are less nutritious.

Fruits: Choose those richest in vitamins, such as strawberries, blueberries, peaches, mangoes, and apples. Limit fruit juices—they are high in sugar and lack fiber—and select 100 percent real fruit juice without added sugar when you do buy juices.

Grains: Select whole or multigrain flours and products; also brown rice, oatmeal, and whole-wheat pasta. Strive to eliminate white bread, white rice, and white pasta from your house.

Meats and Beans (protein): Meats and poultry should be lean with fat and skin removed; fish, eggs, beans, tofu, and other soy foods should be baked, steamed, grilled, or stir-fried, not fried.

Dairy: Low-fat products are preferred, but check with your doctor about serving your child either no-fat or whole-fat products.

Oils: Olive oil is preferred, but safflower and vegetable oils are alternatives.

Fats and Sweets: Limit your child's intake of sugary foods, soda, fried and fast foods.

So, have we answered the question to your satisfaction? Although well-nourished children may not *need* a multi-mineral/vitamin dietary supplement, it is likely the most inexpensive, simple, and effective way to help ensure they are getting the nutrients they need and to support their still-developing immune systems. Overall, most children can benefit from a multimineral/vitamin dietary supplement designed for young bodies, plus an omega-3 essential fatty acid.

If your child has health problems, he or she may need additional or different supplementation, or a therapeutic dose for a limited amount of time to support the immune system and to enhance the natural healing process. You are encouraged to discuss the use of additional vitamin and mineral use beyond a multi-mineral/vitamin with your physician or nutritionist.

Does Your Child Need Individual Supplements?

Individual nutritional supplements are typically given for one of two reasons: a deficiency needs to be corrected, or symptoms or an ailment need to be treated. In either case, you may want to check with your doctor before giving your child an individual supplement, especially if he or she has a medical condition and/or is taking any type of medication or other supplements.

Several nutrients top the list of those that parents worry that their child is not getting in adequate amounts. Here is a brief look at those nutrients.

• **Iron:** A deficiency of this mineral is not as common as it used to be in children and teens, mostly because breakfast cereals and breads are fortified with iron. However, if you have any reason to believe your child may need iron, consult your physician. Children who are very picky eaters or who eat nutritionally inadequate diets may be at risk of iron deficiency, which can cause anemia and impact brain function. Adolescent girls who have begun menstruation may be at increased risk for iron deficiency. Before you give your child iron supplements, however, you should have his or her iron levels checked by a physician. Taking too much iron and/or taking iron supplements when there is no deficiency can be harmful to your child's health.

• **Fluoride:** The American Academy of Pediatrics and other organizations recommend that children use fluoridated toothpaste, even if they live in an area that provides fluoridated drinking water (unless the water contains more than 1.2 milligrams [mg] per liter). Too much fluoride can discolor the teeth and be toxic. The benefit of adequate fluoride is that it is proven to reduce the incidence of cavities. So before you consider giving your child sodium fluoride supplements, make sure you know how much fluoride is in your drinking water. Your local water company should provide that information to you, or you can buy a water testing kit. If your water is not fluoridated, talk to your doctor about how much fluoride your child may need to take.

• **Calcium:** This mineral is the number one additional nutritional supplement that parents buy for their children. A sufficient intake of calcium is critical during childhood up through early adulthood because this is when bones reach their peak mass. If peak bone mass is not reached during these developing years, the risk for osteoporosis is greatly increased later in life. Many vitamin and multivitamin/mineral supplements contain calcium, but it may not be enough.

Children ages one through 10 need 800 mg daily, and those 11 through 18 need 1,200 mg. Children rarely reach these goals through diet alone.

- **Vitamin D:** The need for vitamin D goes hand-in-hand with the calcium requirement, because without sufficient vitamin D, calcium will not be absorbed and utilized properly to build bone. Children older than six months need 400 International Units (IU) of vitamin D daily. Because vitamin D is produced in the skin after exposure to sunlight, children who get exposure to the sun regularly may not need a supplement. Most children's vitamins provide enough vitamin D, but check the label.

- **Omega-3 fatty acids:** Fish oil supplements provide omega-3 fatty acids, which are needed for proper development of the nervous system, brain, heart, and skin. Children who eat fish and nuts regularly are likely to get enough of this critical nutrient, but those who do not could benefit from a high-quality fish oil supplement. One concern about fish oil supplements is contamination with mercury and other toxins, so look for products from companies with high purity standards.

- **Other supplements:** Additional vitamins, minerals, and other nutrients may be helpful to treat specific symptoms and ailments, as we discuss in Part 2.

GIVING YOUR CHILD NUTRITIONAL SUPPLEMENTS

Convincing an older child to take supplements is usually not a problem, but young children may view a supplement as they would a lima bean: yuk! Fortunately, some children's vitamin and mineral supplements are available in fruit-flavored chewables, which are fine for children who are old enough and who agree to chew them. Children younger than four or five years will need to get their supplements in more creative ways. The following tips are for younger children or for older ones who may resist chewing or swallowing a supplement, who have difficulty swallowing tablets or capsules, or who have learning or cognitive disabilities and can benefit from an easier approach to taking supplements.

- Crush tablets and pour out the contents of capsules so the supplement can be mixed into a child's favorite beverage or some food. This may require some experimenting until you get the right balance of supplement with food or beverage so your child does not taste the supplement, which may be bitter or have some other disagreeable taste. Do not use hot foods or beverages to hide the supplement. Some suggestions are applesauce, pineapple or apple juice, jam, or mashed banana.

- Put the supplement into a small portion of food or beverage, and as soon as the child consumes it, "chase" it with something that tastes good. Fresh fruit (pureed or chunks) or fruit juice usually work well. Do not "contaminate" the child's entire portion of food or beverage with the supplement. If you do and the child refuses to or does not finish the portion, he or she will not get the supplement.

- Consider liquid supplements. However, because the liquid preparations tend to lose their potency rather quickly once they have been opened, store them in the refrigerator and make sure the caps are on tight.

- When choosing a chewable vitamin C tablet, get the nonacidic ascorbate form. This is easier on tooth enamel than the common ascorbic acid form of the vitamin.

As a precaution, have your child rinse his or her mouth with water after chewing either form (nonacidic or acidic). In fact, it is a good habit for your child to rinse after chewing any supplement to remove any residual materials that could harm the teeth.

The one thing you do *not* want to do is lead children to think of nutritional supplements as "candy," even though the supplement you give them may look and taste like it. If your

DOSING OF NUTRITIONAL SUPPLEMENTS FOR CHILDREN

- When giving your child nutritional supplements, whether it is a multi-supplement or a single nutrient product, buy supplements that are made specifically for children.

- If you cannot find children's supplements, talk to your pediatrician or other knowledgeable professional about the proper dose for your child.

- As a general rule, dosing of nutritional supplements for children for therapeutic purposes is one-quarter to one-half the stated adult dose, depending on the age and weight of the child.

- Because each child is unique (a 10-year-old child may weigh as much as a 13-year-old child, and vice versa), you should always consult your child's pediatrician before giving him or her nutritional supplements, either as a daily supplement or to prevent or treat a specific condition.

child asks questions about the supplement and seems to need some kind of reassurance or explanation before he or she will take it, you might tell them that the supplement is a very special treat that is good for their body but that it should only be taken once a day. In all cases, supplements should be treated as medicine and so kept out of reach of children.

HOW TO CHOOSE NUTRITIONAL SUPPLEMENTS

You are standing in front of shelves or sitting in front of your computer looking at webpages of supplements, and you are feeling overwhelmed and confused. Dozens of manufacturers produce scores of supplements aimed at children, and all of them claim to have a wonderful product. Regardless of whether you are looking for a general multi-mineral/vitamin supplement or specific individual nutrients, you want to look for reputable manufacturers who make high-quality products. These are more often found in nutrition or health food stores. You can consult with your child's physician about which brands are the best to buy, do research on your own, and visit Consumer-Lab.com, a website that evaluates and reports on supplements. Once you have one or more brands in mind, you can shop around for the best prices.

Buying Supplements

First and foremost, children are not little adults; therefore they should not take a multi-mineral/vitamin designed for adults. You should not cut an adult dose in half when it comes to a multi-supplement, because a child's requirement for each individual nutrient is not half of an adult's. (See the table of Recommended Daily Allowances for children and adults in Chapter 3.) You can, however, divide an adult dose of a supplement that contains a single nutrient if dividing it will give you the child's appropriate dose. To make dosing easier for you, we have included both a child's and an adult's dose (when appropriate) for the natural supplements discussed in Parts 2 and 3 on common ailments and natural supplements to treat them.

Children's dietary supplements can be purchased as capsules, tablets, liquids, and chewables, which are especially popular with younger children. A high-quality supplement will provide the Recommended Dietary Allowance (RDA) of the most essential vitamins and minerals and not exceed the tolerable upper limit on any nutrient in the supplement.

According to a report from Consumer Labs, their evaluation of children's multivitamins found that only one brand tested (Flintstones Gummies) did not exceed the tolerable upper levels (UL) for vitamin A as retinol. Taking too much vitamin A as retinol may cause bone problems. That is not to say that there are not other brands of children's multivitamins on the market that are provide all of the nutrients within safe guidelines. The take-home message is to know the tolerable upper limit for each nutrient when you are shopping for vitamins and minerals for your child. When you look at the chart, you will notice that tolerable upper limits have not been identified for all vitamins and minerals at this time.

Another consideration is lead. In 2008, the Food and Drug Administration (FDA) tested 324 multivitamins designed for children and women and found that nearly all the products contained small traces of lead. The good news is that none of the products tested had more than the safe/tolerable levels for lead, which for children younger than six years is 6 micrograms (mcg) daily. Four of the tested products had no traces of lead. Parents are encouraged to consult the FDA list, Consumer Labs, and other resources for information about lead and other concerns regarding nutritional supplements before making a purchase. (Also see Chapter 3 and the section on lead.)

Shop for supplements that do not have additives such as artificial flavorings, colorings, and sweeteners. Also check the labels for anything to which your child may be allergic, such as milk, wheat, eggs, fish, nuts, soy, or other additives. In short, you want supplements that are free of additives, period.

SHOULD YOU GIVE HERBAL REMEDIES TO YOUR CHILDREN?

A growing number of parents are giving herbal remedies to their children for some of the same reasons they are buying vitamins and other nutritional supplements for them. In the case of herbs, however, more often they are taken to help prevent or treat a specific symptom or ailment.

And why not? Plants have been used for millennia to treat a wide range of symptoms and health problems, and today many of our over-the-counter and prescription medications are based on plants. In fact, about one-quarter of the prescription drugs in the United States contain active ingredients that come from plants. Some medications contain active components that have been synthesized from chemicals that are similar to those found naturally in plants.

Most of the drugs in the United States, however, are composed of patented, synthetic ingredients that can bring in big profits if they are successful in the marketplace. The unfortunate reality is that because Nature's products cannot be patented, they are not profitable the way pharmaceuticals are. But that does not mean herbal remedies cannot be effective. Just like medications, sometimes they work, and sometimes they don't. And in most cases, the herbal products are less expensive and cause fewer side effects than conventional medications. Some people like to say that herbs are Mother Nature's way to be gentler to her children.

That said, we must also discuss the fact that herbal products (and nutritional supplements) are not subject to the same scrutiny by the FDA that over-the-counter and prescription medications are, which means consumers must be vigilant when shopping for and using these products. You should always tell your child's physician that you are planning to give your child an herbal supplement. If your doctor does not agree and you want a second opinion, seek out a healthcare provider who is knowledgeable in the area of herbs and nutrition. This will often be a naturopath who can guide your choice of herbs for your child and your family.

Tolerable Upper Intake Levels (UL) for Vitamins

Age (yr)	Niacin (mg/d)[a]	Vitamin b_6 (mg/d)	Folate (mcg/d)[a]	Choline (mg/d)
Infants				
0–0.5	—	—	—	—
0.5–1	—	—	—	—
Children				
1–3	10	30	300	1000
4–8	15	40	400	1000
9–13	20	60	600	2000
Adolescents				
14–18	30	80	800	3000
Adults				
19–70	35	100	1000	3500
>70	35	100	1000	3500
Pregnancy				
≤18	30	80	800	3000
19–50	35	100	1000	3500
Lactation				
≤18	30	80	800	3000
19–50	35	100	1000	3500

Vitamin C (mg/d)	Vitamin A (mcg/d)[b]	Vitamin D (mcg/d)	Vitamin E (mg/d)[c]
—	600	25	—
—	600	25	—
400	600	50	200
650	900	50	300
1200	1700	50	600
1800	2800	50	800
2000	3000	50	1000
2000	3000	50	1000
1800	2800	50	800
2000	3000	50	1000
1800	2800	50	800
2000	3000	50	1000

The UL for niacin and folate apply to synthetic forms obtained from supplements, fortified foods, or a combination of the two.

[b]The UL for vitamin A applies to the preformed vitamin only.

[c]The UL for vitamin E applies to any form of supplemental α-tocopherol, fortified foods, or a combination of the two.

Tolerable Upper Intake Levels (UL) for Minerals

Age (yr)	Sodium (mg/d)	Chloride (mg/d)	Calcium (mg/d)
Infants			
0–0.5	——e	——e	——
0.5–1	——e	——e	——
Children			
1–3	1500	2300	2500
4–8	1900	2900	2500
9–13	2200	3400	2500
Adolescents			
14–18	2300	3600	2500
Adults			
19–70	2300	3600	2500
>70	2300	3600	2500
Pregnancy			
≤18	2300	3600	2500
19–50	2300	3600	2500
Lactation			
≤18	2300	3600	2500
19–50	2300	3600	2500

Phosphorum (mg/d)	Magnesium (mg/d)[d]	Iron (mg/d)[b]
—	—	40
—	—	40
3000	65	40
3000	110	40
4000	350	40
4000	350	45
4000	350	45
3000	350	45
3500	350	45
3500	350	45
4000	350	45
4000	350	45

ᵈthe UL for magnesium applies to synthetic forms obtained from supplements or drugs only.
ᵉSource of intake should be from human milk (or formula) and food only.

Note: An Upper Limit was not established for vitamins and minerals not listed and for those age groups listed with a dash (—) because of a lack of data, not because these nutrients are safe to consume at any level of intake. All nutrients can have adverse effects when intakes are excessive.

HOW TO CHOOSE HERBAL REMEDIES FOR CHILDREN

First and foremost, consult a knowledgeable healthcare provider before you give herbal remedies to children. Also, do your homework: find out all you can about the herbal remedies you are considering for your child. While many herbal remedies are safe and effective for children when given in child-sized doses, others should be avoided in young people. When in doubt, consult an expert.

For example, earlier in this chapter we mentioned that glucosamine makes up 3 percent of the total amount of herbal supplements that parents buy for their children. Our research shows that experts do not recommend giving glucosamine to children because no studies have been done on the impact it may have on growing bones and joints. Therefore the use of glucosamine and its related supplement, chondroitin sulfate, in young people is not recommended.

The majority of common childhood illnesses, for example, colds, flu, ear aches, and diarrhea, originate from viral infections. Although single herbal remedies can be effective in treating these conditions, you will likely also see combination remedies when you are shopping. There are many good antiviral herbal blends on the market that combine, for example, echinacea, goldenseal, ginger, and other herbs, which we discuss in Part 3. Administer these compound remedies as you would a single one: according to body weight.

Finally, if you are the parent of a young child, it may seem like he or she has one cold after another. In fact, children younger than six or so may have eight or more colds per year until their immune system reaches a higher level of maturity. If you can introduce young children to immune-system-boosting herbal teas (see "Herbal Pops") at an early age, you may not only help significantly reduce the number or severity of colds they develop, but you may also help establish an appreciation for herbal remedies and a habit that they can have the rest of their lives—a habit of preventive care.

HERBAL POPS

• Make a strong infusion using herbs of your choice.

• Mix with an equal amount of 100 percent fruit juice. Apple and grape juice work best.

• Pour into ice pop trays and freeze.

These pops are too cold for children who have an earache, but they can be a great way to introduce your child to herbs and provide immune boosters at the same time in a tasty treat!

HOW TO GIVE HERBAL REMEDIES TO CHILDREN

According to the FDA, if a medication is to be given only for children, then it must be studied in the pediatric population. Around the turn of the millennium, only 25 percent of the prescription drugs marketed in the United States had specific, researched information about how to administer the drug to children. By 2008, the FDA reported that an estimated 50 to 60 percent of prescription drugs used to treat children had been studied at least in some part of the pediatric population. Chances that a medication has been studied in children less than one month old are close to zero.

Most medicines that are given to children—both prescription and over-the-counter—have been developed for adults and then given to children even though they have not been studied in children. The situation for herbal remedies is similar. In the case of herbal supplements, the generally accepted dosing guideline for children is calculated in proportion to the adult dose, which is based on a 150-pound adult. Therefore, a

50-pound child may be given one-third the adult dose and a 100-pound child may be given two-thirds the adult dose. This is only a guideline, and parents are encouraged to speak with a knowledgeable healthcare provider before giving any herbal supplements to their children, especially those younger than 12 and/or those who may have a chronic medical condition, such as asthma, type-1 diabetes, or juvenile arthritis.

If you are feeling especially adventurous, you may want to prepare your own herbal tinctures. It isn't hard to do, and because you can make them with glycerin (available in phar-

HOMEMADE HERBAL TINCTURES

Tinctures can be made with 100-proof alcohol (vodka is a good choice) or with glycerin or cider vinegar. Although the latter two will not be as strong as an alcohol-based tincture, they are still effective and are good options for children's remedies. If you use vinegar, warm it up (not hot) before pouring it.

• Choose your fresh herbs and coarsely chop stems, leaves, and/or roots. Flowers can remain whole.

• Place the herbs in a clean, dry glass jar and fill it to the top with the liquid of your choice. The herbs must be completely immersed in liquid.

• Place an airtight lid on the jar, label the jar with the name of the herb and the date, and store it in a dark place for six to eight weeks.

• Strain out the herbs and pour the tincture into clean, dry bottles. Label with the date and ingredients, and you're done!

macies) instead of alcohol, they are a better choice for children.

BOTTOM LINE

Nutritional supplements and herbal remedies for children can help boost their immune system, supplement a less-than-ideal diet, promote growth, help treat common ailments, and contribute to their overall health and well-being.

CHAPTER TWO

Adults and Natural Supplements

You're not a kid anymore! Whether you are a twenty-something, a feisty fiftyish, or edging into your eighties, your nutritional needs and health issues differ from those you had as a child or adolescent. You may be among the 52 percent of adults who already use nutritional supplements as part of their lifestyle, or one of the smaller but growing number (17.7 percent) of adults who, according to the National Center for Complementary and Alternative Medicine, use supplements other than vitamins and minerals, Whether you already take some type of supplement now, want to consider others, or take nothing now and want to learn more, this chapter is a good introduction, as it explores the changing health needs of men and women as they age and the roles that natural supplements and herbs can have preserving and maintaining health and well-being.

ADULT BODY, ADULT NEEDS

During childhood and adolescence, nutrition—including nutritional supplementation—is critical for normal growth and development. As adults, nutrition is still important for promoting health but there is also a shift of focus to reducing the risk of disease and, in many cases, managing one or more symptoms of an ailment or disorder.

Some specific diseases and conditions associated with poor nutrition and lack of physical activity include heart disease, diabetes, high blood pressure, high cholesterol, arthritis, and various autoimmune conditions such as lupus and chronic fatigue. Overweight and obesity are much more prominent in adults than in young people, although both groups have high, unhealthy rates.

More and more, people are realizing that they can avoid or significantly reduce their dependence on prescription and over-the-counter medications and costly medical procedures if they take steps to safeguard themselves and their family by taking basic multimineral/vitamins and/or B-complex supplements to enhance their immune system and protect against disease, and selected nutritional supplements and/or herbal remedies for certain symptoms or ailments. Sometimes nutritional supplements can be used to complement other treatments that a doctor may prescribe, which may allow individuals to significantly reduce or even eliminate medications they are taking.

CHANGING NUTRITIONAL NEEDS DURING ADULTHOOD

There are specific circumstances and times during adulthood when nutritional needs may change from the "norm," which is generally accepted as following the recommendations of the USDA's Food Pyramid and meeting the goals of the RDAs for vitamins and minerals (see Chapter 3). In fact, the USDA has finally realized that the traditional one-sized pyramid does not fit everyone, and so now you can customize a pyramid to fit your own nutritional needs. If you visit www.MyPyramid.gov, you can enter personal information in the "My Pyramid Plan," and the site will present you with a personalized nutrition plan based on your age, sex, and physical activity level.

Because it is not always possible to follow a nutritious diet, no matter how hard you try, most people can benefit from taking a multimineral/vitamin daily. A B-complex supplement may also be helpful. Many people experience varying degrees of stress, for example, but if there are circumstances in your life that place you in a chronic or near chronic state of emotional and/or physical stress, then you might benefit from taking a high-potency B-complex supplement, as the B vitamins have been shown to help the body deal with stress.

Pregnancy and Breastfeeding

A woman's nutritional needs change significantly when she is pregnant or breastfeeding. According to the American College of Obstetricians and Gynecologists, pregnant women should increase their usual servings of various foods to include three to four servings of fruits and vegetables, nine servings of whole grain foods, three servings of dairy, and three servings of protein. Pregnant women should take supplements that have been approved by their healthcare provider, and the supplements should not replace a healthy diet. Although all pregnant women need to make sure they get the proper nutrition, those who have certain health problems or chronic diseases, dietary restrictions, or complications associated with pregnancy are especially in need of supplementations.

Two supplements that virtually all pregnant women need to take are folic acid and iron. Folic acid reduces the risk of neural tube defects in infants by up to 70 percent. To get that protection, medical experts agree that women should begin taking 400 mcg of folic acid daily at least one month before they begin trying to get pregnant and at least 600 mcg daily once they become pregnant. Most prenatal vitamins contain between 600 and 1,000 mcg of folic acid.

A woman's need for iron increases during pregnancy, because the body makes more blood to support the growing fetus. The extra blood can quickly bring down iron levels, and so prenatal supplements or an iron supplement can help fulfill that need. Because taking too much iron can be harmful, talk to your doctor before beginning an iron supplement.

Herbal Supplements, Pregnancy, and Breastfeeding

Although herbs are natural, not all of them are safe to take during pregnancy. The FDA advises pregnant women to refrain from taking herbs until they consult their doctors or midwives. If you are pregnant and have talked to your healthcare providers about taking herbs, it is recommended that you consult a trained herbalist or other knowledgeable professional about your choice of herbs and how much you can take safely. Some herbal remedies may contain ingredients that may prove harmful to the mother and/or the fetus. A few herbs may cause miscarriage, premature birth, uterine contractions, or harm to the fetus.

That's why in most cases, the herb entries in this book state that the remedies should not be taken if you are pregnant or breastfeeding. This does not necessarily mean that the herb has been shown to be harmful. More often than not, it means that no studies have been done to prove its safety. In fact, very few studies have been done to evaluate the effects of herbs on pregnant or breastfeeding women, or on a developing fetus.

ADULTS OF ALL AGES

More than younger people, adults of all ages typically take more medications, have one or more medical or health concerns, and naturally, are experiencing the gradual effects of aging. Therefore their nutritional needs tend to change with time. While everyone's dietary and nutritional needs are different, there are some generalities, which we mention here briefly.

Take vitamin D, for example, which we discuss in Part 3. Adults of any age, but especially those who are older than 60, have dark skin, or who do not get sufficient exposure to sunlight, should take a vitamin D supplement. Numerous research studies show that the majority of adults have low levels or are deficient in vitamin D. This is important because according to the Vitamin D Council, a deficiency of this nutrient is associated with more than a dozen varieties of cancer as well as many conditions that occur in adulthood, including heart disease, hypertension, diabetes, depression, osteoarthritis, osteoporosis, chronic pain, periodontal disease, and more.

Fortunately, a vitamin D deficiency is easy enough to correct. Allowing your body to manufacture vitamin D is the best way: If you can get midday sun exposure for 15 to 20 minutes three times a week (without sunscreen) year round, you are likely getting a sufficient amount of vitamin D. That's because the body manufactures about 10,000 IU vitamin D in response to 20 to 30 minutes of exposure to summertime sun, which is 50 times more than the RDA of 200 IU.

Don't worry if you can't get the recommended amount of sun: Many people cannot on a consistent basis. The solution is to take 5,000 IU daily for two to three months, then take a vitamin D test (25-hydroxyvitamin D test), which you can get as a home kit or ask your healthcare provider to get for you. Then adjust your dosage of vitamin D so that your blood levels of the vitamin are between 50 and 80 ng/mL year round.

If you are a healthy, active adult who usually follows a nutritious diet, a multimineral/vitamin or a B-complex supplement (discussed in Part 3) may be all you need as an "insurance policy" for your immune system. If, however, you have a chronic health condition or an acute or recurring illness or symptoms, then you may need to take specific nutritional supplements to help your body better cope with the condition.

For example, if you have cancer, an autoimmune disorder such as lupus or rheumatoid arthritis, HIV or AIDS, heart disease, diabetes, liver or kidney disease, or respiratory conditions such as asthma or bronchitis, you are more susceptible to infection, especially if you are taking medications that suppress the immune system. In such cases, you should talk to a knowledgeable professional to determine if you have any nutritional deficiencies and about what supplements could best protect your health.

Impact of Medications on Nutrients

Given the high rates of high blood pressure, high cholesterol, diabetes, obesity, heart disease, gastrointestinal problems, back pain, and other ailments and diseases among adults, it is no surprise that many men and women take medications at least part of the time. Some of these medications can change the way the body absorbs or retains certain nutrients. In some cases, use of a drug can lead to a vitamin or mineral deficiency. Here are some of the medication/nutrient interactions of which you should be aware.

- Anti-anginals for heart disease (ex. Norvasc, Procardia): deplete potassium
- Antibiotics (ex. amoxicillin preparations): deplete biotin, vitamin K, possibly B vitamins
- Antidepressants (ex. Prozac, Zoloft): deplete melatonin
- Anti-diabetics (ex. glucophage): deplete folic acid, vitamin B_{12}
- Blood pressure–lowering drugs (ex. Captopril, Vasotec): Deplete zinc
- Bronchodilators (ex. albuterol): deplete magnesium, calcium
- Cholesterol-lowering drugs (ex. Lipitor, Zocor): deplete coenzyme Q_{10}
- Digoxin: depletes magnesium, potassium, thiamin
- Diuretics (ex. Lasix, Hydrodiuril): deplete potassium, magnesium, B vitamins (especially thiamin)
- Estrogen replacement therapy (ex. Premarin, Prempro): depletes vitamin B_6, folic acid, niacin, vitamin C
- Nonsteroidal anti-inflammatory drugs (NSAIDs; ex. ibuprofen, aspirin): deplete folic acid, iron, zinc, vitamin C, and possibly vitamin B_{12}
- Thyroid hormone replacement (ex. Synthroid): depletes calcium; may interfere with iron
- Ulcer/gastric reflux medications (ex. Prilosec): deplete vitamin B_{12}; may decrease absorption of calcium, magnesium, and other minerals

Impact of Diet on Medications

Sometimes it's the other way around: Foods and beverages have a negative impact on medications. Alcohol, for example, interacts with nearly every medication, especially antidepressants and other drugs that impact the nervous system and brain. As a rule, do not consume alcohol when taking any OTC or prescription medication. Here are a few other food and medication interactions of which you should be aware. Always check with your doctor or pharmacist when you begin a new medication to learn if there are any drug/food interactions.

- Theophylline, which is used to treat asthma, contains xanthines, which are also found in coffee, tea, cocoa, and other products that contain caffeine. If you are taking theophylline and also drink a lot of coffee, for example, you could experience toxic effects from the theophylline (e.g., nausea, vomiting, seizures).

- If you are taking heparin, warfarin, or another drug to prevent clotting, eating large amounts of green leafy vegetables high in vitamin K will counteract the effects of the drugs.

- Grapefruit juice interacts with cholesterol-lowering drugs, estrogen, oral contraceptives, many allergy medications, calcium channel blockers, and some psychiatric medications. The juice changes the way the body metabolizes the medications.

- Orange juice decreases the effectiveness of antibiotics. It also should not be consumed when taking antacids that contain aluminum.

- Pectin and other soluble fibers slow down the absorption of acetaminophen, while bran and other insoluble fibers affect digoxin (a heart medication) in the same way.

PROPER NUTRITION FOR OLDER ADULTS

Older adults have some different health and nutrition needs that should be considered when thinking about nutritional and herbal supplements. One major issue is multiple medications. Eighty percent of seniors take two or more prescription medications, including those to treat heart disease, hypertension, cancer, arthritis, depression, and other conditions. As we noted in the previous section, many of these drugs can interfere with proper nutrition: Some reduce or increase appetite, impair the absorption of one or more nutrients, upset the normal function of the digestive system, cause constipation and/or diarrhea, or even make food taste different. Nutritional supplements may be needed to restore nutritional balance or deficiencies, and may even help in the treatment of symptoms. If you or a loved one is taking over-the-counter and/or prescription medications, check with a pharmacist or other knowledgeable health professional who can help you determine whether the medication and nutritional needs are both being met.

Older adults also are more likely to have some physical limitations, such as diminished cough and gag reflexes, and their immune systems are often less able to fight off infections. It is easy to take effective preventive measures against the threat of respiratory, gastrointestinal, and other infections by ensuring they follow a nutritious diet and take a multivitamin/mineral as a precautionary measure. As an added insurance step, drinking selected herbal teas every day, such as green tea or chamomile, can help enhance the immune system.

Helping Older Adults Eat Well

If you are an older adult or you are caring for an aging parent or other elderly individual, there are some factors to be aware of that can help ensure you or your loved ones are getting proper nutrition.

- **Decline in smell and taste.** A diminished sense of smell and taste can prevent people from enjoying their food

and even make them want to stop eating. Try to enhance foods by mixing textures, such as dried fruits in
yogurt, or adding different herbs or sauces.

- **Physical limitations.** Simple activities such as opening
  a jar, peeling fruit, or standing at the stove may be too
  difficult for some people, and so they are unable to
  properly prepare food for themselves. Arthritis, poor
  muscle strength, dizziness, poor balance, and other
  problems need to be recognized and addressed. Assis-
  tive devices, such as jar openers or nonslip cutting
  boards, are available for people who have physical
  limitations.

- **Side effects of medication.** As already mentioned, this
  can be a significant factor, yet it is often missed or
  ignored. Research the side effects of any medications
  you or a loved one are taking and consult your physician or pharmacist.

- **Financial constraints.** Fixed and limited incomes can
  make it difficult or impossible for some older people
  to purchase nutritious food, or even a sufficient amount
  of food. Meals on Wheels or other assistance programs
  may be able to take some of the burden off. Shop for
  nutritionally dense and less expensive foods, such as
  beans, legumes, and brown rice

- **Poor dental health.** If your teeth, mouth, gums, or jaw
  hurt, it can be difficult or painful to chew. Missing
  teeth, ill-fitting dentures or bridges, mouth sores, and
  other dental problems should be addressed and adjust-
  ments made to the diet, if necessary, to ensure older
  adults get the proper nutrition and that they enjoy their
  food. The addition of nutritional supplements, for example, as well as introducing softer foods, nutritional
  smoothies, or other changes can be made.

- **Forgetfulness.** A declining memory or the onset of dementia can disturb an older person's ability to eat healthful foods, to remember how to shop, or to remember to eat their meals. If you are caring for an older person who is not living with you, offer shopping assistance, check their food supplies, ask about their diet, and watch for signs of weight loss.

- **Depression.** Depression and loneliness can make people not want to eat, even if they are otherwise mentally and physically capable of taking care of themselves. Look for signs of sadness; depression is treatable with natural and conventional means, but it is often overlooked or neglected in older adults.

- **Lack of transportation.** Older adults who no longer drive, who are afraid to navigate through heavy traffic, who have physical limitations that make shopping difficult, or who cannot drive in bad weather may not have access to grocery stores. Neighborhood senior food programs and home delivery of groceries may be helpful, or family members and friends could take turns taking the individual shopping.

- **Use of supplements.** Nutritional supplements can be extremely helpful for older adults, but because the ability to metabolize some nutrients changes with age and medications can interact with certain supplements, it is important to make a list of all medications and supplements you or a loved one is taking and to consult a knowledgeable professional before making any changes.

WOMEN (AND MEN) AND THEIR BONES

As people age, but especially among women, there is a real concern about the development of osteoporosis. Women who have not built up strong bones early in life and continued to support their bone health with an adequate amount of calcium, vitamin D, and other essential bone-supporting nutrients run a real risk of getting this bone-thinning disease. Women begin to lose calcium from their bones during and after the onset of menopause at a rate of 1 percent per year for about five years, then the loss rate slows down until they reach age 75 or 80.

Let's not forget the men. The National Osteoporosis Foundation says there are about 2 million men who have osteoporosis, and another 12 million who are at risk. This compares with the 8 million women who have osteoporosis and the 22 million who are at risk. Men get osteoporosis less often and at a later age, mainly because they do not go through menopause, they have higher levels of testosterone, and their bones are generally larger and stronger than a woman's.

Calcium does not work alone. Without enough vitamin D, the body cannot properly absorb and use the calcium. Since the majority of adults in the United States have low or deficient levels of vitamin D, you should evaluate how much calcium and vitamin D you are getting to make sure you are not selling yourself and your bones short. (See Chapter 3 for the RDA for calcium for you and your entire family.)

Experts have determined that calcium from foods is absorbed much better than calcium from supplements. Foods high in calcium include low-fat or no-fat dairy products, as well as foods that are calcium-fortified, including many soy beverages, cereals, breads, and juices. Foods that are naturally rich in calcium and those that have been fortified are generally equally effective in delivery the mineral to the body. However, some calcium-fortified cereals may contain phytate, which can interfere with the absorption of calcium. Also, eating lots of high-fiber foods can contribute to low calcium levels because the presence of lots of fiber in the intestinal tract reduces the absorption of calcium and other nutrients. This does not mean you should shy away from fiber—just that you may need to ensure you are getting enough nutrients if you are eating a high-fiber diet. If you cannot meet the recommended 1,000 mg or more per day through your diet, add a calcium supplement to your routine.

HERBAL REMEDIES FOR ADULTS

A gradually increasing number of adults are turning to herbal remedies both for preventive and treatment purposes. In a study published by the Mayo Clinic in 2007, the researchers questioned more than 30,600 adults about their use of ten different herbs commonly used to treat specific health conditions. The survey was part of the 2002 National Health Interview Survey.

The investigators found that 19 percent of the adults had used herbs within the last year, and of those, 57 percent had used herbs to treat a specific health problem. Among the people who had used only one herb (except echinacea and ginseng), about one-third had taken the herb appropriately (according to results of scientific research) while two-thirds did not. Adults younger than 60 and black adults were significantly less likely to use herbal remedies (with the exception of echinacea) based on scientific evidence. When it comes to echinacea, however, adults tended to take it properly about half the time. What do these study results mean?

Although a significant number of adults are turning to herbal remedies, many of them are not taking them according to evidence-based recommendations. If herbs are not taken as recommended, it can defeat the purpose of taking them: Not only do you risk not getting any benefit from the herb, you also may believe that the herbs are ineffective. Herbal remedies are potent substances, and like medications, their best chance of providing you with the benefits you want relies on your taking the remedy as recommended.

One remedy for failing to take herbs as recommended is to learn more about the remedy you want to take. We recommend that you look them up in this book (see Parts 2 and 3), browse the Internet for scientific studies, talk to a knowledgeable professional. Take the recommended amount (dosages of herbal remedies for adults are calculated on the basis of a 150-pound individual); purchase your herbs from a reputable source, and store them as directed. Heed any warnings about their use, especially if you are pregnant or breast-feeding or taking medications. Herbal remedies can be an important part of your plan to prevent disease and maintain health and well-being.

BOTTOM LINE

Once the growth and development years are behind you, much of your focus needs to be on preventing illness and maintaining health. Attention to nutrition is critical if you hope to achieve these goals. This chapter contains a taste of what you need to know about nutritional and herbal supplements and their relationship to your health during adulthood. Now we bring together some tools you and your family can use to help achieve your health goals naturally.

CHAPTER THREE

The Natural Medicine Survival Plan for Your Family

This chapter provides you with a Natural Medicine Survival Plan for your Family so you can take control of your family's health. This plan consists of four main ingredients: environmental knowledge, trusted healthcare provider(s), an understanding of supplements, and a natural medicine survival kit.

It seems that the old-fashioned medicine cabinet on the bathroom wall is no longer enough: Increasing environmental pollutants, rising healthcare costs, and an overwhelming load of information coming at us from every direction has made it necessary for parents to step back and take stock of their health care and the role they have in it for themselves and their families. Here are a few important tools; use them wisely.

ENVIRONMENTAL FACTORS CAN IMPACT YOUR HEALTH

It has become commonplace to be warned by the news media and other outlets about how yet another environmental pollutant, chemical, or other substance can damage your health. The dangers seem to come from every direction: foods and beverages contaminated by bacteria or other harmful organisms, toys tainted with lead and other dangerous toxins, plastics laced with harmful chemicals, and substances in our water and food that can change how hormones act. What can parents do to protect their children and themselves against the health dangers posed by these substances?

Your best defense is knowledge, which you can use to take the actions necessary to protect your family. Here are some of the more common environmental factors to be aware of and what you can do about their impact.

BISPHENOL A (BPA)

Do you and your family use plastic water bottles or sippy cups? Do you heat food in the microwave in plastic containers? Do you buy food in metal cans? Then you and your family are exposed to bisphenol A (BPA), an industrial chemical that is used to harden plastic.

BPA is a toxic chemical that mimics estrogen, a hormone that controls the reproductive system, brain development, and maturation of the fetus. A growing number of recent studies have shown that BPA can leach into food and beverages and may have a wide range of negative health effects, including:

- Increased risk for heart disease
- Increased risk for asthma in children
- Tendency for aggressive and hyperactive behavior in toddlers
- Increased susceptibility to develop an enlarged prostate and prostate cancer
- Increased risk of neuroblastoma, a cancer that often develops in early childhood
- Birth defects and disruption of normal endocrine function
- Increased risk of breast cancer
- Neurological difficulties with memory, learning, and attention

It's hard to avoid plastic: It's used in everything from cars to baby bottles and furniture. The plastic you need to be most aware of is the kind that contains BPA that can be absorbed by your body and affect your health. Therefore you want to avoid, as much as possible, contact between plastics and your food, beverages, and/or mouth. To protect you and your family against BPA contamination, here are some tips:

- Choose containers that are free of BPA, such as porcelain, stainless steel, or glass.
- Invest in safe, reusable water bottles and mugs.
- Do not heat plastic wrap, baby bottles, or other plastic food and beverage containers.
- Shop for BPA-free baby bottles, pacifiers, and toys.
- Look for the recycling code on plastic bottles and containers. If it has a number 7, it may contain BPA. Safer plastics have the numbers 2, 4, and 5.
- Do not buy acidic foods, such as tomatoes, tomato products, and apple juice, in cans because the acid speeds up the leaching of BPA into the food.
- Ask your dentist if he or she uses BPA-free dental sealants and fillings.

LEAD AND OTHER HEAVY METALS

Exposure to lead and other heavy metals can affect people of all ages, but especially unborn babies and young children. There are 23 heavy metals, and small amounts of them are common in the environment and diet. In fact, small amounts of them are necessary for good health, but large amounts can cause acute or chronic poisoning, including damage to the nervous system, lower energy levels, and damage to the blood and vital organs. Long-term exposure to heavy metals may result in slowly progressing conditions that mimic Parkinson's disease, multiple sclerosis, Alzheimer's disease, and muscular dystrophy.

Of the 23 heavy metals, we will look at three of the more common ones: lead, arsenic, and mercury.

Lead

Each year in the United States, more than 300,000 children ages one to five years old are found to have unsafe levels of lead in their blood, which can cause symptoms ranging from headache to stomach pain, anemia, and behavioral problems. Young people are more likely to experience health hazards due to lead exposure because their smaller, developing bodies are more susceptible to absorbing and retaining the toxic metal.

One of the main ways children are exposed to lead is old paint in older homes. Old paint tends to peel easily, and children will often put the pieces into their mouths. Although paint no longer is made with lead, buildings with walls and ceilings painted before the late 1970s likely have lead paint. Another source of lead is in some toys, usually those made in China. These are typically recalled by the Food and Drug Administration as soon as the toxin is discovered, so parents should be alert to recalls. Less common sources of exposure are water contaminated by corroding lead pipes, contaminated soil, and food that has been stored in containers glazed with lead or in lead-lined cans.

If you have any reason to believe your child may have been exposed to lead, either by being inhaled or swallowed, talk to your doctor about getting a simple blood test, as many children with lead poisoning do not show any symptoms or the symptoms are mistaken for something else. Symptoms of lead poisoning may include irritability or behavioral problems, pica (eating odd things such as dirt and paint chips), difficulty concentrating, headaches, weight loss, loss of appetite, fatigue, constipation, pale skin (from anemia), metallic taste in the mouth, and abdominal pain.

A variety of health problems are associated with lead poisoning. Once lead gets into the body, it can be distributed anywhere. In the blood, for example, it can damage red blood cells and cause anemia. Lead poisoning can also cause other problems in children, including:

- Decreased bone and muscle growth
- Damage to the nervous system and kidneys
- Damage to hearing
- Speech and language problems
- Poor muscle coordination
- Developmental delays
- Seizures and unconsciousness (at extremely high levels)

Arsenic

While lead is a common cause of acute heavy metal poisoning in children, arsenic is the equivalent culprit in adults, because the main source of contamination is the workplace and hazardous waste sites. Arsenic is released into the environment mainly by the smelting process of copper, lead, and zinc, as well as by the manufacture of glass and chemicals. The manufacture of pesticides releases arsine gas, which contains arsenic. Arsenic is also found in water supplies, which contaminates fish, as well as in paints, fungicides, and wood preservatives. This heavy metal attacks the blood, kidneys, central nervous system, digestive system, and skin.

Mercury

Mercury finds its way into the body through several routes. Coal-burning power plants are the largest human-caused source of mercury released into the air in the United States, along with burning hazardous waste, producing chlorine, and spilling mercury. The mercury in the air eventually contaminates water and land, and it is changed into methylmercury, a highly toxic form that accumulates in fish, shellfish, and animals that eat fish. When people eat fish that are contaminated with mercury, they risk the consequences of mercury poisoning.

Both short-term and long-term exposure to mercury can lead to serious health problems in anyone, but the EPA and the FDA especially warn women of childbearing age, women who are pregnant or breastfeeding, and young children to be careful about the types of fish and shellfish they eat and how often they eat it. See "Fish and Mercury," below, for the fish typically lowest in mercury.

Other possible sources of mercury contamination include vaccines and dental fillings. Both of these sources are controversial. Many individuals believe that vaccines are associated with autism while the courts determined in March 2010 that mercury is not to blame. Leakage of mercury from dental fillings is frequently named as the cause of symptoms associated with mercury poisoning, although the American Dental Association insists these fillings are safe.

Among fetuses, infants, and children, the main effect of methylmercury poisoning is impaired neurological development, with negative effects on cognitive thinking, memory, attention, language, and fine motor and visual spatial skills. Methylmercury exposure can also cause muscle weakness, impaired peripheral vision, pins and needles, and problems with walking.

FISH AND MERCURY

Low Mercury Content
Canned light and white tuna
Cod
Flounder
Haddock
Halibut
Herring
Pollock
Salmon
Shellfish

Medium to High Content
Bass
King Mackerel
Shark
Swordfish
Tilefish
White Perch

PHTHALATES

Phthalates (pronounced *fal'-ates*) are a group of industrial chemicals used to make plastics like polyvinyl chloride (PVC) more flexible, and also as solvents. These chemicals are also known as endocrine disruptors because they mimic the body's hormones and have been shown to cause reproductive and neurological damage in animal tests. Plastics are such a large and important part of our society, and phthalates are equally ubiquitous, yet they are not typically identified on labels. So phthalates can be found in items ranging from food packaging to hoses, shower curtains, detergents, nail polish, shampoo, toys, air fresheners, and vinyl flooring, yet chances are you will never see a label that identifies phthalates as an ingredient or component. This can make it difficult to avoid phthalates when you want to . . . and you want to.

That said, here are a few ways you can identify phthalates in some products by their chemical names or abbreviations.

- BzBP (benzylbutyl phthalate) is found in car products, personal care products, and flooring.
- DBP (di-n-butyl phthalate) and DEP (diethyl phthalate) are often ingredients in personal care products such as shampoos, hair gels, body lotions, perfumes, cologne, and deodorants.
- DEHP (di-(2-ethylhexyl) phthalate or Bis (2-ethylhexyl) phthalate) is used in PVC plastics and some medical devices. It has been classified as a probable human carcinogen by the EPA and as a potential carcinogen by the Department of Health and Human Services.
- DMP (dimethyl phthalate) is found in insect repellents and some plastics.
- If you see the word "fragrance," it may denote a combination of ingredients, possibly including phthalates.
- Plastics that have the recycling number 1, 2, or 5 are much less likely to contain phthalates; avoid numbers 3 and 7.

Research in animals has shown that phthalates can reduce sperm counts and cause testicular atrophy and structural deformities in the reproductive system. Studies in humans have suggested that phthalates are associated with symptoms of ADHD and behavioral problems in young children. Children may consume more than an average amount of phthalates if they chew on toys or teethers that are made of phthalate-softened vinyl. The other common way to get phthalates is through food, when the chemical has leached into foods from their packaging or containers, similar to the way BPA enters food (see "Bisphenol-A").

In 2008, the US Congress passed legislation that banned six phthalates (DEHP, DBP, BBP, DINP, DIDP, and DnOP) from children's toys and cosmetics. In addition, several major retailers, including Evenflo, Gerber, Lego, Toys-R-Us, and Wal-Mart, began to phase out phthalate-contaminated toys. Other phthalates and other sources of the chemical remain in the environment.

XENOESTROGENS

Xenoestrogens are substances in the environment that, once they are ingested, inhaled, or absorbed into the skin, act like estrogen and can cause levels of the hormone to rise in the body. This creates a condition known as estrogen dominance, which can happen in people of any age, both females and males. In young girls who have been exposed to xenoestrogens, some have begun to menstruate as early as age five or six. In young males, it can cause breast enlargement. Many other symptoms and ailments are associated with estrogen dominance (as shown in the following table).

SIGNS AND SYMPTOMS OF ESTROGEN DOMINANCE

Accelerated aging

Allergies

Anxiety

Breast cancer (women
    and men)

Decreased sex drive

Depression

Dry eyes

Endometriosis

Fatigue

Fibrocystic breasts

Gallbladder disease

Hair loss

Headaches

Infertility

Insomnia

Irregular menstrual
    periods

Magnesium deficiency

Mood swings

Osteoporosis

PMS

Thyroid dysfunction

Zinc deficiency

How are we exposed to xenoestrogens? You don't have to look far: They are lurking in your home, school, workplace, and in the world at large right now. Some of the places xenoestrogens can be found include:

- Commercially-raised, nonorganic meats and dairy products
- Laundry detergent (use baking soda, white vinegar, trisodium phosphate instead)
- Fabric softeners and dryer sheets (use white vinegar)
- Soaps, shampoos, body lotions, and cosmetics that contain phenoxyethanol or paraben (read labels)
- Hormone replacement therapy (use natural, bio-identical hormones)
- Air fresheners that contain phthalates
- Insecticides (dieldrin, DDT, endosulfan, heptachlor, lindane, methoxychlor)
- Sunscreen lotions (look for 4-methylbenzylidene camphor)
- Pesticides
- Weedkillers (atrazine)
- Caffeine

Another important way to steer clear of xenoestrogens is to avoid reheating food in plastic or Styrofoam containers, because the xenoestrogens leach out of the plastic. Instead, use glass or ceramics to store and heat or cook food and water. Even though you may not reheat fast food that comes in Styrofoam containers, it is best to avoid this type of packaging (and in most cases, the food inside!) because it is not healthy for you and your family.

FOOD ADDITIVES

More than 14,000 man-made chemicals are added to food products in the United States. In a majority of cases, these are not substances that Nature intended people to consume, although some additives (e.g., sodium chloride, also known as table salt) are essential for life, even though they should be consumed in limited amounts. Infants begin taking in additives the moment they have their first breastfeeding: If the mother eats food that contains additives, then her infant is exposed as well.

Not all food additives are dangerous to your health, although many are considered to be "questionable" or have been shown to cause cancer or other health problems in animals but not in people. Some additives are especially problematic for individuals who are allergic or sensitive to the substances.

Although we cannot discuss all the questionable or hazardous food additives, here is a list of some of the more common and harmful ones. Check food labels for these additives when making food purchases.

- **Acesulfame K:** This is a sugar substitute also known as Sunette or Sweet One. It is often an ingredient in chewing gum, dry mixes for beverages, instant tea and coffee, gelatin desserts, puddings and non-dairy creamers. Acesulfame K has caused cancer in animals.

- **Artificial colorings:** The majority of artificial colorings added to foods are synthetic dyes. Some have been banned already, but others are still being added to food and are suspected of being carcinogenic or toxic. Examples include blue 1 and 2, red 3 and 40, and yellow 5 and 6.

• **Aspartame:** This sugar substitute is available as Equal and NutraSweet. Aspartame contains the amino acid phenylalanine. One out of 20,000 infants is born without the ability to metabolize this substance, and if it reaches high levels in the blood it can cause mental retardation. In addition, some people experience dizziness, headache, seizures, and menstrual problems after ingesting aspartame.

• **BHA and BHT:** These chemicals are often added to foods to prevent oxidation and retard rancidity. BHA has been named as possibly carcinogenic to humans by the International Agency for Research on Cancer, and California has listed it as a cancer-causing substance.

• **Caffeine:** Caffeine is found naturally in coffee, tea, and cocoa, but it is also added to many beverages, including so-called "energy" drinks. Caffeine promotes the secretion of stomach acid, can temporarily elevate blood pressure, and may dilate some blood vessels while constricting others. For some people, caffeine is mildly addictive and causes headaches if they stop drinking caffeinated beverages. Caffeine in small amounts typically does not cause a problem for most people, but children and pregnant women should avoid it.

• **Monosodium glutamate (MSG):** Many people think of MSG as the additive in Chinese food, but it is found in many more foods. MSG enhances the flavor of food, which is why manufacturers use it, but it can cause headache, tightness in the chest, dizziness, nausea, and other symptoms in people who are sensitive. MSG can appear as other ingredients in foods, including but not limited to hydrolyzed vegetable protein, yeast extract, textured protein, malt extract, autolyzed yeast, sodium caseinate, and calcium caseinate.

- **Nitrates and nitrites:** These closely related chemicals are used to preserve meats, such as bacon, luncheon meats, hot dogs, and sausages. Nitrate converts to nitrite, which combines with compounds called secondary amines to form nitroamines, which can cause cancer. Even if processed meats did not contain these chemicals, they still typically have a high-fat, high-sodium content, which is reason enough to avoid them.

- **Olestra:** Imagine you pick up a food item and the warning label says "This Product Contains Olestra. Olestra may cause abdominal cramping and loose stools. Olestra inhibits the absorption of some vitamins and other nutrients. Vitamins A, D, E, and K have been added." Does this food sound appetizing? This is the warning that the FDA at one time required manufacturers to put on food items that contain this fake fat that has no calories, cholesterol, or fat. Although the FDA eventually removed the labeling requirement, that did not change the fact that Olestra causes these symptoms and has that effect on nutrients. The side effects can occur after eating even small amounts of the snacks.

- **Potassium bromate:** This additive is used to increase the volume of bread. Bromate causes cancer in animals, and the additive has been banned nearly everywhere in the world except the United States and Japan. In California, bread that contains potassium bromate must carry a cancer warning label.

- **Sulfites:** These chemicals were once used to keep cut fruits and vegetables looking fresh, to prevent dried fruits from becoming discolored, and to prevent discoloration, bacterial growth, and fermentation in wine. After many reports of allergic reactions to sulfites, including several deaths, the FDA banned the chemicals from most fruits and vegetables. However, sulfites are still used in fresh-cut potatoes, dried fruits, and wine. Sulfites can worsen asthma symptoms, cause hives, and trigger other allergic reactions.

FINDING A TRUSTED HEALTHCARE PROVIDER

Whether you are looking for a doctor for yourself or one for your children, you need a professional you can trust, who you can communicate with, who is accessible, and who seems to understand your and your family's needs. Everyone has their own healthcare and insurance issues to deal with, which may limit your choices. However, even if your choice of doctors is restricted to a certain number or area, exercise as much freedom of choice as you can. Whether you are looking for a general practitioner, a pediatrician, a naturopath, or a specialist, the process is basically the same. So, here are some general questions and factors to consider when choosing a personal physician or other healthcare provider. See the Appendix for a list of organizations you can contact to find healthcare providers in your area.

Questions to Ask When Choosing a Physician

- Where did the doctor attend medical school?

- When and where did the doctor do residency?

- Does the doctor have a specialty that is relevant to your family?

- Is the doctor knowledgeable about nutrition and/or herbal remedies?

• With which hospital is the doctor affiliated?

• Does the doctor have a solo or group practice? Would you be required to see this doctor's associates if he or she is not available? Do you have information on these other associates?

• Is the doctor available or reachable after hours and on weekends?

• Does the doctor have lab or x-ray facilities in the office?

• Is the office conveniently located?

• Will the doctor be caring for more than one family member?

• Do you know any of this doctor's other patients? It is good to speak with other patients if possible.

• Is this doctor active in the community? Some physicians give talks or lectures in the community. If so, attend so you can evaluate him or her in action

• Does the doctor visit his/her patients in the hospital or nursing facilities?

• Have there been any disciplinary actions against the doctor? You can check with your state's medical board or with Consumer Checkbook (www.checkbook .org/doctors/discipline.cfm), a nonprofit reporting agency. Most states provide the information free of charge.

Things to Consider When Choosing a Naturopath or Herbalist

• Only seven schools in North America license individuals for a Doctor of Naturopathy degree, which requires three years of standard premedical education followed by four years of naturopathic medicine training in acupuncture, botanical medicine, counseling, homeopathic medicine, nutrition, and psychology. Do not accept credentials from a naturopath who has attended any school other than these seven: Boucher Institute of Naturopathic Medicine (Vancouver); National University of Health Sciences (Chicago, IL); National College of Naturopathic Medicine (Portland, OR); Bastyr University (Seattle, WA); Southwest College of Naturopathic Medicine (Tempe, AZ); Canadian College of Naturopathic Medicine (Toronto); and University of Bridgeport College of Naturopathic Medicine (Bridgeport, CT).

• Naturopathic medicine is not regulated in most states, which means people can call themselves naturopaths even if they do not meet the standards of the profession. The states that license naturopaths are Alaska, Arizona, California, Connecticut, Hawaii, Idaho, Kansas, Maine, Minnesota, Montana, New Hampshire, Oregon, Utah, Vermont, and Washington, as well as the District of Columbia, the US Virgin Islands, and Puerto Rico.

• Some naturopaths specialize in one or more areas, such as nutrition or herbal medicine. Some cater to children or the elderly. Ask for the naturopath's specialty.

• Naturopaths do have some limitations. For example, they usually do not have hospital privileges, although they typically will make referrals. Not all states grant prescription privileges to naturopaths, so check with your state's guidelines. Naturopaths also do not perform surgery or handle trauma such as burns, heart attacks, and fractures.

• Herbalists are not licensed or certified by states, although there are organizations for professional herbalists that can help you find a practitioner in your area. See the Appendix for a list of herbalist organizations.

UNDERSTANDING THE WORLD OF NUTRIENTS AND HERBS

The realm of nutritional and herbal supplements has its own terminology, and it helps to be familiar with the more common terms so you can make informed decisions when choosing supplements for you and your family. Here is an introduction to some of those terms.

Vitamin and Mineral Terms

RDA (Recommended Daily Allowance) is a term that has been used for decades to rate vitamins. However, it is gradually being replaced by a new standard called the dietary reference Intake (DRI). The DRI was created to shift the focus of why we should take supplements. In the past, the emphasis was on preventing a vitamin or mineral deficiency, but now the DRI focuses on lowering the risk of chronic diseases, such as cardiovascular disease. The DRI values fall into four categories. As parents, you should be especially interested in the first two.

• RDA is the current rating on most vitamins.
• UL (tolerable Upper intake Level) is the maximum dose likely to be safe in 98 percent of the population. If you or your child takes any nutrient in an amount that exceeds the UL, it may result in serious health

problems, which vary depending on the nutrient.
- AI (Adequate Intake) is the amount that experts use if there is insufficient data to calculate the RDA.
- EAR (Estimated Average Requirement) is the amount that meets the nutritional requirements of 50 percent of the population.

On the following pages are tables for the RDAs and ULs for all ages. You can refer to these figures as a guide when choosing nutritional supplements.

Herbal Remedy Terms

Herbal medicines are available in several forms and have certain characteristics. One form is a tincture, which you can make yourself at home, as we explained in Chapter 2. Here are some other terms you may encounter in this book and when shopping for or reading about herbal remedies.

- Astringent: Herbs that increase the firmness and tone of tissues and reduce the mucous discharge from the nose, vagina, and wounds.
- Decoction: A tea made by boiling herbs for an extended time (typically 10 minutes or longer). Decoctions are most often made from the roots, bark, stems, or hard seeds of herbs.
- Diuretics: Herbs that increase the flow of urine.
- Emetics: Herbs that induce vomiting.
- Emollients: Herbs that soothe and soften when applied topically.
- Expectorant: Herbs that help excrete mucus from the lungs and throat.
- Extracts: Herbal extracts are made by using a solvent like alcohol or water to remove the active components from the leaves, root, bark, or flowers of an herb. The liquid extract is then concentrated using evaporation to produce a powder, which can be used to make capsules and tablets.

DIETARY REFERENCE INTAKES (DRIs):
Recommended Intakes for Individuals, Vitamins

Life Stage Group	Vit A (mcg/d)[a]	Vit C (mg/d)	Vit D (mcg/d)[b,c]	Vit E (mg/d)[d]	Vit K (mcg/d)	Thiamin (mg/d)	Riboflavin (mg/d)
Infants							
0–6mo	400*	40*	5*	4*	2.0*	0.2*	0.3*
7–12mo	500*	50*	5*	5*	2.5*	0.3*	0.4*
Children							
1–3y	300	15	5*	6	30*	0.5	0.5
4–8y	400	25	5*	7	55*	0.6	0.6
Males							
9–13y	600	45	5*	11	60*	0.9	0.9
14–18y	900	75	5*	15	75*	1.2	1.3
19–30y	900	90	5*	15	120*	1.2	1.3
31–50y	900	90	5*	15	120*	1.2	1.3
51–70y	900	90	10*	15	120*	1.2	1.3
>70y	900	90	15*	15	120*	1.2	1.3
Females							
9–13y	600	45	5*	11	60*	0.9	0.9
14–18y	700	65	5*	15	75*	1.0	1.0
19–30y	700	75	5*	15	90*	1.1	1.1
31–50y	700	75	5*	15	90*	1.1	1.1
51–70y	700	75	10*	15	90*	1.1	1.1
>70y	700	75	15*	15	90*	1.1	1.1
Pregnancy							
14–18y	750	80	5*	15	75*	1.4	1.4
19–30y	770	85	5*	15	90*	1.4	1.4
31–50y	770	85	5*	15	90*	1.4	1.4
Lactation							
14–18y	1,200	115	5*	19	75*	1.4	1.6
19–30y	1,300	120	5*	19	90*	1.4	1.6
31–50y	1,300	120	5*	19	90*	1.4	1.6

Food and Nutrition Board, Institute of Medicine, National Academies

Niacin (mg/d)[e]	Vit B$_6$ (mg/d)	Folate (mcg/d)[f]	Vit B$_{12}$ (mcg/d)	Pantothenic Acid (mg/d)	Biotin (mcg/d)	Choline[g] (mg/d)
2*	0.1*	65*	0.4*	1.7*	5*	125*
4*	0.3*	80*	0.5*	1.8*	6*	150*
6	0.5	150	0.9	2*	8*	200*
8	0.6	200	1.2	3*	12*	250*
12	1.0	300	1.8	4*	20*	375*
16	1.3	400	2.4	5*	25*	550*
16	1.3	400	2.4	5*	30*	550*
16	1.3	400	2.4	5*	30*	550*
16	1.7	400	2.4[i]	5*	30*	550*
16	1.7	400	2.4[i]	5*	30*	550*
12	1.0	300	1.8	4*	20*	375*
14	1.2	400[i]	2.4	5*	25*	400*
14	1.3	400[i]	2.4	5*	30*	425*
14	1.3	400[i]	2.4	5*	30*	425*
14	1.5	400	2.4[h]	5*	30*	425*
14	1.5	400	2.4[h]	5*	30*	425*
18	1.9	600[j]	2.6	6*	30*	450*
18	1.9	600[j]	2.6	6*	30*	450*
18	1.9	600[j]	2.6	6*	30*	450*
17	2.0	500	2.8	7*	35*	550*
17	2.0	500	2.8	7*	35*	550*
17	2.0	500	2.8	7*	35*	550*

Note: This table (taken from the DRI reports, see www.nap.edu) presents Recommended Dietary Allowances (RDAs) in **bold type** and Adequate Intakes (AIs) in ordinary type followed by an asterisk (*). RDAs and AIs may both be used as goals for individual intake. RDAs are set to meet the needs of almost all (97 to 98 percent) individuals in a group. For healthy breastfed infants, the AI is the mean intake. The AI for other life stage and gender groups is believed to cover needs of all individuals in the group, but lack of data or uncertainty in the data prevent being able to specify with confidence the percentage of individuals covered by this intake.

[a]As retinol activity equivalents (RAEs). 1 RAE = 1 mcg retinol, 12 mcg β-carotene, 24 mcg α-carotene, or 24 mcg β-cryptoxanthin. The RAE for dietary provitamin A carotenoids is twofold greater than retinol equivalents (RE), whereas the RAE for preformed vitamin A is the same as RE.

[b]As cholecalciferol. 1 mcg cholecalciferol = 40 IU vitamin D.

[c]In the absence of adequate exposure to sunlight.

[d]As α-tocopherol. α-tocopherol includes *RRR*-α-tocopherol, the only form of α-tocopherol that occurs naturally in foods, and the *2R*-stereoisomeric forms of α-tocopherol (*RRR*-, *RSR*-, *RRS*-, and *RSS*-α-tocopherol) that occur in fortified foods and supplements. It does not include the *2S*-stereoisomeric forms of α-tocopherol (*SRR*-, *SSR*-, *SRS*-, and *SSS*-α-tocopherol), also found in fortified foods and supplements.

[e]As niacin equivalents (NE). 1 mg of niacin = 60 mg of tryptophan; 0–6 months = preformed niacin (not NE).

[f]As dietary folate equivalents (DFE). 1 DFE = 1 mcg food folate = 0.6 mcg of folic acid from fortified food or as a supplement consumed with food = 0.5 mcg of a supplement taken on an empty stomach.

[g]Although AIs have been set for choline, there are few data to assess whether a dietary supply of choline is needed at all stages of the life cycle, and it may be that the choline requirement can be met by endogenous synthesis at some of these stages.

[h]Because 10 to 30 percent of older people may malabsorb food-bound B_{12}, it is advisable

for those older than 50 years to meet their RDA mainly by consuming foods fortified with B_{12} or a supplement containing B_{12}.

ᶠIn view of evidence linking folate intake with neural tube defects in the fetus, it is recommended that all women capable of becoming pregnant consume 400 mcg from supplements or fortified foods in addition to intake of food folate from a varied diet.

ᵍIt is assumed that women will continue consuming 400 mcg from supplements or fortified food until their pregnancy is confirmed and they enter prenatal care, which ordinarily occurs after the end of the periconceptional period—the critical time for formation of the neural tube.

- Infusion: A tea made by steeping herbs in freshly boiled (but not still boiling) water for five to 20 minutes. This approach is most often used for less hardy parts of the plant, including the flowers and leaves, and for plants that contain volatile oils that would be lost in the steam if they were boiled.
- Sedatives: Herbs that help calm the nervous system.
- Stimulants: Herbs that assist in the function of the body, increasing energy.
- Tincture: This remedy is made by soaking an herb in grain alcohol (vinegar or wine also can be used) for a specified amount of time, depending on the herb. The solution is then strained, leaving behind the tincture.
- Tonics: Herbs that increase energy levels and strengthen the body. They are often referred to according to the part of the body they are aiding; for example, heart tonics, liver tonics.

YOUR HOME NATURAL MEDICINE SURVIVAL KIT

Minor symptoms and illnesses can happen at any time, especially when there are children in the house. You can be prepared by having a well-stocked and current natural medicine chest on hand to handle everything from indigestion to minor cuts and bruises and the sniffles. You will want to customize your personal natural medicine chest to meet your family's specific needs. Be sure to check for any expiration dates on items in your medicine chest so you can avoid a 2 AM run to the all-night pharmacy for a remedy just when you need it the most.

- Adhesive tape to secure bandages and dressings
- Antiseptic cream to prevent infection associated with minor cuts and scrapes
- Aloe vera plant (you can keep this on your windowsill or in your garden), for minor burns, sunburn, minor abrasions, and other skin irritations

DIETARY REFERENCE INTAKES (DRIs):
Recommended Intakes for Individuals, Elements

Life Stage Group	Calcium (mg/d)	Chromium (mcg/d)	Copper (mcg/d)	Fluoride (mcg/d)	Iodine (mcg/d)	Iron (mg/d)	Magnesium (mg/d)
Infants							
0–6mo	210*	0.2*	200*	0.01*	110*	0.27*	30*
7–12mo	270*	5.5*	220*	0.5*	130*	**11**	75*
Children							
1–3y	500*	11*	340	0.7*	90	7	80
4–8y	800*	15*	440	1*	90	10	130
Males							
9–13y	1,300*	25*	700	2*	120	8	240
14–18y	1,300*	35*	890	3*	150	11	410
19–30y	1,000*	35*	900	4*	150	8	400
31–50y	1,000*	35*	900	4*	150	8	420
51–70y	1,200*	30*	900	4*	150	8	420
>70y	1,200*	30*	900	4*	150	8	420
Females							
9–13y	1,300*	21*	700	2*	120	8	240
14–18y	1,300*	24*	890	3*	150	15	360
19–30y	1,000*	25*	900	3*	150	18	310
31–50y	1,000*	25*	900	3*	150	18	320
51–70y	1,200*	20*	900	3*	150	8	320
>70y	1,200*	20*	900	3*	150	8	320
Pregnancy							
14–18y	1,300*	29*	1,000	3*	220	27	400
19–30y	1,000*	30*	1,000	3*	220	27	350
31–50y	1,000*	30*	1,000	3*	220	27	360
Lactation							
14–18y	1,300*	44*	1,300	3*	290	10	360
19–30y	1,000*	45*	1,300	3*	290	9	310
31–50y	1,000*	45*	1,300	3*	290	9	320

Manga-nese (mg/d)	Molyb-denum (mcg/d)	Phos-phorus (mg/d)	Sele-nium (mcg/d)	Zinc (mg/d)	Potas-sium (g/d)	Sodium (g/d)	Chloride (g/d)
0.003*	2*	100*	15*	2*	0.4*	0.12*	0.18*
0.6*	3*	275*	20*	3	0.7*	0.37*	0.57*
1.2*	17	460	20	3	3.0*	1.0*	1.5*
1.5*	22	500	30	5	3.8*	1.2*	1.9*
1.9*	34	1,250	40	8	4.5*	1.5*	2.3*
2.2*	43	1,250	55	11	4.7*	1.5*	2.3*
2.3*	45	700	55	11	4.7*	1.5*	2.3*
2.3*	45	700	55	11	4.7*	1.5*	2.3*
2.3*	45	700	55	11	4.7*	1.3*	2.0*
2.3*	45	700	55	11	4.7*	1.2*	1.8*
1.6*	34	1,250	40	8	4.5*	1.5*	2.3*
1.6*	43	1,250	55	9	4.7*	1.5*	2.3*
1.8*	45	700	55	8	4.7*	1.5*	2.3*
1.8*	45	700	55	8	4.7*	1.5*	2.3*
1.8*	45	700	55	8	4.7*	1.3*	2.0*
1.8*	45	700	55	8	4.7*	1.2*	1.8*
2.0*	50	1,250	60	12	4.7*	1.5*	2.3*
2.0*	50	700	60	11	4.7*	1.5*	2.3*
2.0*	50	700	60	11	4.7*	1.5*	2.3*
2.6*	50	1,250	70	13	5.1*	1.5*	2.3*
2.6*	50	700	70	12	5.1*	1.5*	2.3*
2.6*	50	700	70	12	5.1*	1.5*	2.3*

Note This table presents Recommended Dietary Allowances (RDAs) in **bold type** and Adequate Intakes (AIs) in ordinary type followed by an asterisk (*). RDAs and AIs may both be used as goals for individual intake. RDAs are set to meet the needs of almost all (97 to 98 percent) individuals in a group. For healthy breastfed infants, the AI is the mean intake. The AI for other life stage and gender groups is believed to cover needs of all individuals in the group, but lack of data or uncertainty in the data prevent being able to specify with confidence the percentage of individuals covered by this intake.

Sources: *Dietary Reference Intakes for Calcium, Phosphorous, Magnesium, Vitamin D, and Fluoride* (1997); *Dietary Reference Intakes for Thiamin, Riboflavin, Niacin, Vitamin B_6, Folate, Vitamin B_{12}, Pantothenic Acid, Biotin, and Choline* (1998); *Dietary Reference Intakes for Vitamin C, Vitamin E, Selenium, and Carotenoids* (2000); *Dietary Reference Intakes for Vitamin A, Vitamin K, Arsenic, Boron, Chromium, Copper, Iodine, Iron, Manganese, Molybdenum, Nickel, Silicon, Vanadium, and Zinc* (2001); and *Dietary Reference Intakes for Water, Potassium, Sodium, Chloride, and Sulfate* (2004). These reports may be accessed via http://www.nap.edu.

B-COMPLEX SUPPLEMENT

This is an example of the dosage ranges available in typical average- to high-potency B-complex supplements. Each manufacturer has its own formula, and you should consult with your physician about which potency is best for you and each member of your family. Generally, children ages four to 12 take one-half the adult dose, beginning at the low end of the ranges. Children older than 12 can take the adult dose. Consult your physician about giving a B-complex supplement to children ages four years and younger.

Vitamin	Dosage Range
Thiamin	25 to 100 mg
Riboflavin	25 to 100 mg
Niacin/niacinamide	50 to 100 mg / 10 to 30 mg
Vitamin B_5	50 to 200 mg
Vitamin B_6	25 to 100 mg
Folic acid	200 to 400 mcg
Biotin	200 to 1,500 mg
Vitamin B_{12}	50 to 100 mcg
Choline	25 to 100 mg
Inositol	25 to 100 mg
Para-aminobenzoic acid	10 to 50 mg

NOTE: No daily values have been established for choline, inositol, and para-aminobenzoic acid.

- Baking soda for skin irritation, insect bites, sunburn, heartburn
- Bulb syringe to remove nasal secretions in babies and toddlers
- Disposable gloves

- Echinacea extract for cold and flu symptoms
- Ginger tea for nausea
- Hydrogen peroxide to disinfect minor cuts and scrapes
- Multi-minerals/vitamins for children and adults
- Neti pot for clearing congested nasal passages due to cold, flu, allergies, etc. (usually comes with dry saline solution packets)
- Probiotics for nausea, indigestion, diarrhea, constipation, colic, and ear infections
- Sharp scissors (with rounded ends)
- Sterile pads and gauze
- Syrup of Ipecac to induce vomiting in case of accidental poisoning
- Thermometer (age-appropriate)
- Triangular bandages for support
- Tweezers for removing splinters and other foreign objects
- Zinc lozenges

BOTTOM LINE

If you arm yourself with some basic tools, you can feel more secure about taking care of yourself and your family's health needs. An understanding of natural supplements and herbal remedies, a knowledge of environmental factors that can impact your health, a healthcare provider you can trust, and a natural medicine survival kit can help provide that feeling of security.

PART II

Common Ailments That Can Affect You and Your Family

From colic to arthritis, the common cold to PMS, this section looks at some of the more common ailments that can affect you and your family, from infancy through the senior years, and some of the nutritional supplements and herbal remedies you can take to help prevent and treat them. We have focused on conditions for which there are nutritional and herbal methods that have been shown to be effective.

Remember, similar to over-the-counter and prescription medications, nutritional supplements and herbal remedies may work for some people and not for others. A person's personal and medical history, biochemistry, and lifestyle habits have an impact on his or her response to preventive and treatment approaches. Each of the entries covered in this chapter provides you with an opportunity to explore natural options and to have more control over your health and that of your family. Once you find a supplement that interests you, turn to Part 3 to learn more about it and how it is used.

Before taking any new supplement, consult with a knowledgeable healthcare professional.

ACNE

If you have a teenager and he or she does not have acne, you have one lucky kid. Between 80 and 95 percent of adolescents develop acne *(acne vulgaris)*, a chronic inflammatory skin condition that is characterized by lesions—white heads, black heads, cysts, abscesses, and other red and/or inflamed eruptions. These lesions usually appear on the face and neck, but they can also develop on the back, chest, upper arms, and shoulders.

Acne is not just the bane of adolescents: About 6 percent of men and 8 percent of women older than 24 years experience outbreaks of the condition as well. Overall approximately 17 million people in the United States deal with this problem at some point in their lives.

Causes and Symptoms

Do chocolate bars and French fries cause acne? No, say the experts, although fatty foods and those high in sugar can promote the condition once you have it. Research now shows that hormone imbalances (typical of the teen years and around menopause), family history, stress, and a weakened immune system have been named as probable culprits.

Acne occurs when hair follicles become clogged with sebum, an oily substance that is made by the oil glands attached to the follicles. Normally, sebum travels through the follicles and reaches the skin, where it can be washed away. For people who have acne, however, the sebum mixes with cells that the follicles shed, and the mixture blocks the pathway to the skin's surface. Once the follicles are completely filled up, they erupt and deposit sebum, cells, and bacteria on the skin, which irritates it and causes lesions to form.

How Supplements Can Help

- Aloe vera gel can be applied to painful outbreaks of acne and provide effective relief. One study found that 90 percent of acne lesions healed completely with aloe vera within five days of application.

- The B vitamins can help promote healthy skin. A high-potency B-complex supplement taken daily may help. Children and adolescents should take an age-appropriate B-complex supplement.

- MSM can help clear up acne. The suggested dose is 1,000 to 2,000 mg daily. Once the acne has significantly improved, you can reduce the dose by half. This dose is safe for children age six years and older.

- Tea tree oil is an antibacterial and can be applied to acne three times daily and then before bedtime to be left on overnight. Use a solution of 5 percent tea tree oil after thoroughly cleaning the area to be treated. Apply with a cotton swab.

- Zinc supplements have been shown to improve acne. A zinc-sulfate-hydrate supplement (10 milliliters [mL]) taken three times a day for several days can be followed by 50 mg daily of zinc picolinate for up three months. Because this dose can deplete copper levels in the body, it is recommended that you also take 2 to 3 mg copper daily while using zinc at these dosages.

Children older than 10 years can take one-half these suggested doses, with their doctor's knowledge. There should be no need to treat children younger than 10 years for acne.

When to See a Doctor

Occasionally acne can develop into a more serious problem. If the skin around the lesions is hot and red, this indicates cystic acne, which requires medical treatment. Acne that is accompanied by fever and boils could be acne fulminans, which also requires immediate treatment.

ALLERGIC RHINITIS/HAY FEVER

Allergic rhinitis is an allergic reaction that affects at least 20 percent of Americans of all ages. The reactions occur when the immune system overreacts to usually harmless substances, called allergens, that people inhale. The two types of allergic rhinitis are seasonal allergic rhinitis (hay fever) and perennial allergic rhinitis, which occurs all year. Hay fever is caused by outdoor allergens, such as pollen, ragweed (the most common outdoor allergen), and fungus, while perennial allergic rhinitis is caused by indoor allergens such as pet dander, mold, and dust mites.

Causes and Symptoms

Although allergic rhinitis is a common condition, experts do not know exactly why the body has such a negative reaction to certain substances. This is what they do know: When a person is exposed to an allergen, a whole cascade of events gets started. First the body reacts by producing an antibody, called immunoglobulin E (IgE), to bind the allergen. The antibodies then attach to a type of blood cell called mast cells, which are found in the airways and other sites in the body. The allergens bind to the IgE, which is attached to the mast cell, which then prompt the mast cells to release chemicals into the bloodstream. The main chemical, histamine, is the one that causes most of the symptoms of an allergic reaction.

And what are those symptoms? You allergy sufferers know them well: itchy and watery eyes, sneezing, itchy and runny nose, itchy roof of the mouth, and sometimes a sore throat and headache as well.

How Supplements Can Help

- Butterbur has been shown in at least two studies to reduce symptoms of hay fever and asthma. Suggested dose is 500 mg daily for adults. Pregnant and breast-feeding women should not take butterbur. For children ages six to 12 years, one-quarter to one-half the adult dose can be effective. Begin with the lower dose. For children older than 12 years, one-half to the full adult dose is suggested.

- Garlic juice is effective in resolving symptoms of hay fever. You can crush garlic cloves and extract 1 teaspoon of fresh juice and take it twice daily for seven days. Symptoms typically resolve in six to eight hours after taking the juice. Children typically do not like this remedy. However, if you can mix it into their food, use one-third the amount for children who weigh 50 pounds or two-thirds for those weighing 100 pounds.

- NAC helps the body make glutathione, a potent antioxidant that can help with allergies. The suggested dose is 200 mg three times daily for adults. Children ages six to 12 may take one-quarter the dose; ages 12 and older, one-half.

- Quercetin, a potent bioflavonoid, has both antiallergy and antihistamine properties, which makes it a good candidate for treating allergies. The suggested dose is

100 mg three times daily for adults; talk to your doctor about doses for children 12 years and older.

- Stinging nettle is a popular remedy for allergic rhinitis. Until recently, there was little scientific evidence that it was effective, but a 2009 study in *Phytotherapy Research* identified the compounds in this herb that inhibit allergic and other inflammatory responses. Suggested dose is 300 mg one to two times daily for adults. It is not recommended for pregnant women. Suggested doses for children are one-quarter the adult dose for children age six years and younger, and one-half the adult dose in children older than six years.

When to See a Doctor

Hay fever usually doesn't require attention from a doctor unless treatment options are not providing significant relief or you or your child develop a painful cough or difficulty breathing. Because severe or recurrent hay fever symptoms may reduce your resistance to respiratory conditions, you should contact your physician if the symptoms persist.

ARTHRITIS

More than 47 million adults and 300,000 children in the United States have been diagnosed with some form of arthritis. Although there are more than 100 forms of arthritis, the vast majority of affected individuals have either osteoarthritis (about 27 million) or rheumatoid arthritis (1.3 million). Gout affects approximately 3 million people, and because it is treated differently than these other two main types of arthritis, we cover it in a separate entry. Among children, juvenile rheumatoid arthritis is the most common. (Because there are no natural supplements or herbal remedies recommended for treating juvenile rheumatoid arthritis, we do not cover this condition.)

Both osteoarthritis and rheumatoid arthritis are chronic

conditions. Osteoarthritis is commonly called the "wear-and-tear" arthritis, because it involves the wearing away of the joint's cartilage. The breakdown of cartilage causes the bones to rub against each other. Osteoarthritis typically affects certain joints, including the hips, hands, lower back, neck, and knees, and mostly affects people age 40 years and older.

Rheumatoid arthritis is an autoimmune condition, which means the body attacks its own tissues. In this disease, the immune system responds by causing inflammation of the lining (synovium) of the joints, which can lead to long-term joint damage. Rheumatoid arthritis usually develops in people between the ages of 30 and 50, but it can start at any age.

Causes and Symptoms

The causes of osteoarthritis are not known, but certain factors increase the risk of getting the disease, including family history, being overweight, joint injury, lack of physical exercise, nerve injury, aging, and repeated overuse of certain joints. Symptoms include joint pain, stiffness, and loss of movement in the affected joints.

Experts are not certain why the body attacks its own tissues in rheumatoid arthritis. Some people with the disease have high levels of an antibody called rheumatoid factor, which may cause the immune system to malfunction in some people. Not everyone who has rheumatoid arthritis has a high rheumatoid factor, and not everyone who has a high factor has the disease. Other risk factors for rheumatoid arthritis include being female (women are two to three times more likely to get the disease) and genetics. Some experts believe rheumatoid arthritis may be caused by an infection.

Rheumatoid arthritis progresses in three stages. At first, there is swelling of the synovial lining, which causes pain, stiffness, redness, warmth, and swelling around the affected joint. During the second stage, the synovium thickens, and during the third, the inflamed cells release enzymes that may break down bone and cartilage, which causes the affected joint to lose its shape and alignment, resulting in more pain and loss of movement. Because rheumatoid arthritis is a systemic condition (affects the entire body), other symptoms may include fatigue, low-grade fever, inflamed eyes, and loss of appetite.

How Supplements Can Help

Note: All of the dosages given here are for treatment of arthritis in adults.

- Devil's claw: For inflammation and pain associated with arthritis, the suggested dose is one that provides at least 50 mg of harpagosides daily. Look for a standardized extract and take 100 to 200 mg one to two times daily.

- Feverfew: This herb can help reduce inflammation. Suggested dose: 125 mg daily of standardized to 0.2 percent parthenolide taken once to twice daily.

- Glucosamine and chondroitin: The suggested dose of glucosamine is 500 mg three times daily before meals. You can take this dosage for up to six months, then you should reduce it to between 500 and 1,000 mg daily. Some healthcare providers recommend also taking chondroitin along with glucosamine. If you do, the ratio should be 5:4; that is, if you take 500 mg glucosamine, you would take 400 mg chondroitin. Sometimes glucosamine is also taken with MSM (see "MSM").

- Omega-3 fatty acids: Research shows that taking omega-3 supplements for up to three months can improve morning stiffness and joint pain in people who have rheumatoid arthritis. Suggested dose: 1,000 to 3,000 mg daily. Do not take more than 3,000 mg daily because of a risk of bleeding.

- SAM-e (s-adenosyl-L-methionine) can relieve pain from osteoarthritis, but you will likely need to take the supplement for at least one week before you notice significant benefits. Suggested dose: 600 to 1,200 mg daily.

When to See a Doctor

Consult a doctor if your joints become inflamed or infected or if your joint pain is accompanied by a fever.

ASTHMA

Asthma is a chronic respiratory condition in which certain factors trigger a response in the air passages, causing them to become constricted and thus restrict the flow of air in and out of the lungs. According to the National Health Interview Survey (2008), more than 23 million Americans have asthma, and 7 million of them are children. Because children have smaller airways than adults, asthma can be especially serious for them. Asthma is the number one cause of chronic illness among children in the United States. Although it can begin at any age, most children show their first symptoms by age five.

Causes and Symptoms

The exact cause of asthma is not known, but experts believe it is probably a combination of environmental and genetic factors. What they do know is that people with asthma are hypersensitive to one or more triggers, which may include a long list of items such as allergy-type irritants (e.g., pollen, dust, mold, pet dander), environmental pollutants (e.g., cigarette smoke, perfumes, air fresheners, chemical irritants, air pollution), certain foods, strenuous exercise, or stress. Symptoms of asthma include tightness in the chest, wheezing, breathing difficulties, and coughing, which are the result of inflamed airways and muscle spasms of the airways, which then increase the production of mucus.

How Supplements Can Help

- Butterbur has been shown to reduce bronchial spasms in asthma patients. A suggested adult dose is 50 to 75 mg twice daily. Children may be given one-third to two-thirds of the adult dose, based on their body weight.

- Ginkgo may interfere with the protein in the blood that contributes to spasms of the airways. A suggested dose is 60 to 250 mg of standardized ginkgo extract once daily. Children may start at the low end of the suggested dosage range, however, you should consult your doctor before giving this herb to a child who has asthma.

- Magnesium is a natural bronchodilator, which means it can relax the bronchial passages that lead to the lungs. The suggested dosage is 500 mg magnesium citrate or magnesium aspartate daily for adults. Studies of magnesium for asthmatic children have focused on intravenous magnesium; therefore, you need to consult your physician before giving magnesium supplements to children.

- Omega-3 fatty acids are known for their ability to reduce inflammation, which can be most helpful in asthma patients. Taking omega-3s daily may help ward off what is known as late-phase inflammation, which is the inflammation that occurs up to 24 hours after an acute asthma attack and sticks around for weeks. A suggested initial dose is 1,000 mg of fish oil or flaxseed oil daily, which can be increased to 3,000 to 6,000 mg in adults depending on symptoms. You should consult your doctor before starting omega-3 supplements, especially in children, to get the optimal dosage.

- A combination of omega-3 (1,000 mg), zinc (15 mg), and vitamin C (200 mg) was found to be effective in relieving asthma symptoms in children. The study, which was published in *Acta Paediatrica* in April 2009, showed that this combination of supplements improved lung function and inflammation.

When to See a Doctor

If your asthma attacks have increased in frequency and/or severity, if you are having difficulty controlling your attacks, or if your medications are not providing sufficient relief, consult your physician. Let him or her know if you are taking supplements or herbal remedies, as they can have an impact on your medication.

ANEMIA

"Anemia" is a general term for a number of conditions in which the number and/or size of red blood cells is changed in some way, which causes an insufficient amount of oxygen to reach the tissues. It is not known exactly how many people suffer from anemia, but certain populations are more likely to have it than others.

For example, according to the National Anemia Action Council, anemia affects 10 percent of people older than 65, 17 to 41 percent of people who have inflammatory bowel disease, 20 percent of pregnant women, 30 to 60 percent of people who have rheumatoid arthritis, and 80 percent of chemotherapy patients. Anemia can also affect children, who usually have iron deficiency anemia (see below).

Generally, people who have anemia experience fatigue, dizziness, headache, insomnia, poor appetite, stomach discomfort, or chest pain. Specific types of anemia also are associated with specific symptoms.

Causes and Symptoms

Although there are several types of anemia, they all share certain characteristics; namely, they involve red blood cells, oxygen, and hemoglobin. Red blood cells require iron, folic acid, vitamins B_{12} and C, protein, and copper to stay healthy. A major function of red blood cells is to transport oxygen via a substance called hemoglobin. Healthy red blood cells can carry 200 to 300 hemoglobin molecules, but when something causes the number of red blood cells or hemoglobin molecules to decline, the result is anemia. Here are a few of the more common types of anemia.

- Iron-deficiency anemia. This is the type most people think of when anemia is mentioned. This type usually occurs when people do not get enough iron from their diet (the main reason children get this type of anemia), they do not absorb iron properly, or they have lost a lot of blood. Children can develop iron-deficiency anemia from drinking too much cow's milk, as it does not contain much iron and actually hinders absorption of iron. Pregnancy and heavy menstrual flow can also cause iron-deficiency anemia. In addition to the symptoms already mentioned, individuals may be pale and have a sore tongue and dry, brittle nails. Children who have iron-deficiency anemia may develop learning disabilities and behavior problems.

- B_{12}-deficiency anemia. This type is found most often in people who have conditions that interfere with the absorption of nutrients, such as celiac disease or Crohn's disease. Additional symptoms may include tingling in the arms and legs, yellowish skin, and weight loss.

- Folic acid deficiency anemia. This type is most often seen in the elderly and in pregnant women, as both populations have a greater need for the vitamin. The main contributors to folic acid deficiency anemia are stress, poor diet, and absorption problems.

- Inherited forms of anemia. These include sickle cell anemia, in which the red blood cells have abnormal shapes, and thalassemia, in which hemoglobin production is abnormal.

How Supplements Can Help

The supplements you take will depend on the type of anemia you need to treat.

- The B vitamin folic acid is a remedy for anemia caused by a deficiency of this nutrient. A suggested dose is 400 mcg two to three times daily, one-quarter to one-half this dose for children age six years and older.

- Dandelion improves the body's ability to absorb iron from food and supplements. Suggested dose is 5 to 10 mL of tincture taken in water three times daily. For children, base the dose on the child's weight. If the child weighs 50 pounds the dose would be one-third the adult dose; at 100 pounds, two-thirds the adult dose.

- Iron-deficiency anemia can be treated with iron supplements. A typical dose for adults is 100 mg daily; however, taking too much iron can be dangerous, so you should consult your doctor before starting supplementation. The iron supplement that is most gentle on the stomach is ferrous peptonate. If you cannot find this form, then ferrous chelate and ferrous gluconate are also suggested. Children typically need to receive 8 to 10 mg daily of iron, but you should consult your physician before giving your child an iron supplement because too much of the mineral can be toxic.

- Vitamin C should be taken along with iron supplements, because it boosts the absorption of iron. Dose: 500 mg daily for adults; one-quarter to one-half this dose for children age six years and older.

• Vitamin B_{12} is recommended for anemia associated with a deficiency of this nutrient. Suggested dose is 1,000 to 2,500 mcg twice daily for adults, one-quarter to one-half this dose for children age six years and older.

When to See a Doctor

If you have symptoms of anemia, you should consult a doctor to get a definite diagnosis. This is especially important if you are pregnant or elderly or if you have a medical condition that affects your ability to absorb nutrients.

ATHLETE'S FOOT

The medical term for this annoying condition is tinea pedis, and it isn't even limited to athletes. In fact, up to 70 percent of the population has athlete's foot at some point in their lives. Athlete's foot is common among adolescents and adults, but not so much among children. If your feet begin to itch and you see white, scaly patches between your toes or on the bottom and sides of your feet, you may have athlete's foot.

Causes and Symptoms

The culprits behind athlete's foot are fungi called dermatophytes, which thrive in close, damp environments, like between your toes in tight shoes or damp socks. Plastic shoes are especially good breeding grounds for the fungi. Athlete's foot is contagious and can be spread from person to person by direct, skin-to-skin contact, or from objects to humans, such as in public locker rooms, saunas, swimming pool areas, and showers, but also from contaminated floors, rugs, and clothing. Sometimes the fungi are spread from animals (usually household pets) to humans.

Symptoms of athlete's foot can include itching and burning and may be mild to severe. In severe cases the skin may crack and bleed, and tiny sores and blisters may form, causing pain. In mild cases some people don't have any symptoms at all.

How Supplements Can Help

- Aloe vera gel can relieve itching and redness. Apply the gel to the affected areas twice daily until the symptoms clear. This treatment can be used for children and adults.

- Garlic fights fungal infections. You can either rub a crushed clove of garlic on the affected area or, if this burns, you can dilute fresh garlic oil (you can make your own by crushing garlic cloves) with olive oil and apply to the affected areas once or twice a day.

- Ginger is a strong antifungal agent. Boil a cup of water, add 1 ounce of chopped fresh ginger, and simmer for 20 minutes. Let the tea cool and apply to your feet twice daily. This approach is safe for both adults and children.

- Tea tree oil is a powerful antifungal agent. To use tea tree oil, place 10 drops into a quart of warm water and soak your feet for ten minutes twice daily for ten days. After each soaking, dry your feet thoroughly and apply tea tree oil to the affected areas with a cotton swab. Continue to apply the tea tree oil twice daily for at least two months after the ten days of soaking. This approach can be used for children and adults. If the 100 percent tea tree oil irritates your skin, dilute it 50/50 with aloe gel or vitamin E oil.

When to See a Doctor

Athlete's foot typically clears up without a doctor's intervention, but if you have sores or blisters that have opened up and become infected, you may need an antibacterial medication.

ATTENTION DEFICIT HYPERACTIVITY DISORDER

Attention deficit hyperactivity disorder (ADHD) is one of the most common childhood disorders, and it can continue through the teen years and adulthood. Approximately 8 percent of children and adolescents have ADHD, while about half as many (4.1 percent) adults ages 18 to 44 have ADHD. Symptoms in adults are generally milder than those in children and adolescents.

The initial onset in children is usually by age three years, but the condition is generally not diagnosed before the age of six or seven. Three to five times more boys than girls have ADHD.

Causes and Symptoms

Several theories have been proposed as to what causes ADHD. Genes are believed to play a significant role, although experts tend to agree the condition arises from a combination of factors. Those include environmental factors (e.g., cigarette smoking and/or alcohol use during pregnancy), poor nutrition (e.g., sugar, food additives), social environment, and brain injuries.

The main symptoms of ADHD are difficulty staying focused and paying attention, hyperactivity, great impatience, difficulty processing information, and difficulty controlling behavior (e.g., blurting out inappropriate comments, difficulty sitting still). To be diagnosed with ADHD, a child must have symptoms for six months or longer and to a degree greater than is seen in other children of the same age.

How Supplements Can Help

Both children and adults can be treated the same way for this condition. Here are some suggestions.

- B-complex supplements can work one of two ways. One, they can reduce your child's level of hyperactivity, but on the flip side, they may also increase the activity level, in which case you can give selected B vitamins individually to avoid such an increase. The following B vitamins can be helpful: B_6 at 10 mg daily, B_1 at 20 mg daily, and folic acid at 400 mcg daily for children age six years and older.

- Magnesium supplements may be helpful if your child complains of stomachaches, muscle pain, headaches, or has trouble with sleep. These symptoms often indicate a deficiency of magnesium. Children with ADHD can be magnesium deficient because the high adrenaline level associated with hyperactivity causes them to eliminate excessive amounts of magnesium in their urine. A suggested dose is 100 mg daily for younger children and 200 mg for those age 12 and older, taken at bedtime. If your child's diet is low in calcium, you should add a calcium supplement as well: 400 mg for younger children and 800 for older children and adults.

- Omega-3 fatty acids in the form of fish oil can be beneficial, as many children with ADHD have low levels of essential fatty acids, which have a crucial role in preserving nerve function in the brain. A suggested dose for children is 500 mg and for adults 1 g of fish oil with a ratio of 3:2 for EPA and DHA, respectively. You can increase the dose gradually until you see results, but do not exceed 3 g daily, as too much fish oil can raise the risk of bleeding. (See the "Omega-3 Fatty Acids" entry in the Supplement section for an explanation of how fish oil supplements are determined.)

- Pycnogenol can prevent and reduce free radical damage to the brain and nerve tissue. Some experts believe it may improve the function of important neurotransmitters (dopamine and norepinephrine) in the brain. Pycnogenol can also improve the delivery of magnesium and zinc to the brain and reduce stress hormone levels. Research shows that taking 1 mg of pycnogenol per 2.2 pounds of body weight can reduce hyperactivity and improve motor-visual coordination and concentration. Talk to your doctor before initiating treatment with pycnogenol for your child.

- Zinc can be helpful in reducing hyperactivity, impulsiveness, and impaired socialization. The dose used in research in children is 40 mg daily. Any long-term use (longer than one month) of zinc should be balanced with copper: 0.5 mg for younger children, 1 mg for adolescents, and 2 mg for adults.

When to See a Doctor

Parents should take their child to a physician if he or she shows signs and symptoms of ADHD so an accurate diagnosis can be made. Also, if your child is not responding to treatment or seems to be getting worse, contact your doctor as soon as possible.

BRONCHITIS

Bronchitis can sneak up on you: it starts like a common cold but then you develop symptoms that leave you feeling washed out. In most cases, bronchitis is caused by viruses, although a small percentage of episodes are bacterial. Two forms of bronchitis can develop: acute bronchitis, which usually follows a bout with the common cold or flu and then resolves in about a week; and chronic bronchitis, which hangs on for months. Bronchitis affects people of all ages, and it occurs often. Approximately 8 million Americans suffer with chronic bronchitis each year, and more than 14 million experience an acute case of the infection.

Causes and Symptoms

Viral bronchitis is often caused by the same viruses that cause the flu, influenza A and B. Several bacteria, including *Mycoplasma pneumoniae,* also cause bronchitis. The infection attacks the bronchial tubes, which carry air to your lungs. Infected tubes swell and fill up with mucus, which makes breathing difficult. People who smoke, have asthma, a weakened immune system, or who are repeatedly exposed to lung irritants are more susceptible to bronchitis.

Symptoms of bronchitis include a wet or dry cough, chest pain, wheezing, burning in the chest, fever with chills, fatigue, and a rattle in the throat. Both adults and children can get bronchitis, and the symptoms are similar for both. Infants, however, typically get bronchiolitis, which involves the smaller airways and causes symptoms similar to asthma.

How Supplements Can Help

- Butterbur has been shown to reduce bronchial spasms in people with bronchitis. A typical adult dose is 50 to 100 mg twice daily with meals. Children ages six to 12 years may take one-quarter to one-half the adult dose; children 12 and older may take one-half to the full adult dose.

- Echinacea stimulates the immune system to fight the infection. Typical dosage is 300 mg capsules three times daily or up to 60 drops of tincture three times daily. Do not take echinacea for longer than two weeks. Children who weigh 50 pounds can take one-third the adult dose; those who are 100 pounds can take two-thirds the adult dose.

- Garlic is both an expectorant and an antibacterial fighter. Look for garlic capsules or tablets standardized to contain 0.6 percent allicin and take a dose that will give you 4,000 mcg of allicin daily (typically up to three 500 mg capsules daily). For children, dosing is typically one-third to two-thirds of the adult dose, depending on the child's weight. Consult your healthcare provider if you want to treat your child with garlic for this condition.

• Magnesium: Taking this supplement can ease wheezing and other respiratory complaints. Naturopaths commonly recommend taking 300 to 600 mg daily. Children older than six years can take one-quarter to one-half this dose.

• Stinging nettle: Try this herb as a tea: 2 teaspoons of dried herb per 8 ounces of boiling water. Steep for 5 to 10 minutes. Enjoy 2 to 3 cups daily. Children who weigh 50 pounds may have 1 cup daily; at 100 pounds, 2 cups.

When to See a Doctor

If you have a fever and your symptoms have lasted for more than seven to 10 days, the bronchitis may have developed into pneumonia. Contact your physician immediately. Other symptoms that should prompt you to call your healthcare provider include shortness of breath, change in the color of the mucus, and coughing up greater and greater amounts of mucus.

BREAST CANCER

The words "breast cancer" are frightening to most women. It seems that every woman knows someone who has the disease, and in far too many instances, they have it themselves. Breast cancer is the second most common form of cancer in women, surpassed only by nonmelanoma skin cancer. According to the American Cancer Society, it is also the second leading cause of cancer death in women, exceeded only by lung cancer.

Not all breast cancer is the same; it can be invasive or noninvasive, and there are several different types within each category. For example:

- Invasive ductal carcinoma is the most common type of breast cancer, representing 80 percent of invasive breast cancers. It begins in a duct and then can spread beyond the breast.

- Invasive lobular carcinoma begins in the milk-producing glands and can spread to other parts of the body. It represents about 10 percent of invasive breast cancers.

- Ductal carcinoma in situ is a noninvasive type of breast cancer and the most common of this type. It starts in and stays within the ducts. It represents about 20 percent of all new cases of breast cancer.

- Lobular carcinoma in situ begins in and stays in the lobules.

In 2009, an estimated 192,370 new cases of invasive breast cancer and 62,280 new cases of noninvasive breast cancer were diagnosed. More than 40,000 women died of the disease. And we did not forget the men. Approximately 2,000 men are diagnosed with breast cancer each year, and about 20 percent die of the disease. The good news is that death rates from breast cancer have been declining, and women can take steps to help prevent and treat this disease using natural supplements.

Causes and Symptoms

Breast cancer develops when certain changes (mutations) occur in the DNA that trigger normal breast cells to become cancerous. In a small percentage of cases, the mutations are inherited and thus increase the risk that a woman will develop breast cancer. Two examples are mutations of the tumor suppressor genes named BRCA1 and BRCA2.

Most breast cancer, however, develops when changes that have not been inherited occur in breast cells during a woman's life. Experts have identified risk factors for breast cancer, and most of them are things women can do something about. They include being overweight, drinking alcohol, smoking, eating a high-fat diet, going through menopause after age 55, never having children, using birth control pills, and having a first child after age 35. The risk of getting breast cancer also increases as women get older.

The first clue that a woman could have breast cancer may be the presence of a tumor as seen on a mammogram or thermogram. Some women find a lump during a breast self-exam, which is a sign to see their physician as soon as possible. Women should consult their healthcare providers if they notice any of the following symptoms:

- a change in the normal appearance of the breast, such as a change in size, shape, color, and/or feel of the skin
- retraction of the nipple
- swelling of the breast
- discharge from the nipple, either clear or bloody
- sudden breast pain or tenderness

The most common symptom of male breast cancer is a painless lump in the breast. Sometimes there is nipple discharge, nipple retraction, or ulceration of the skin.

How Supplements Can Help

Along with making lifestyle changes suggested by the risk factors, here are some nutritional and herbal supplements that may help prevent breast cancer or complement conventional treatment and thus improve quality of life.

- A high-potency B complex supplement should be taken along with folic acid, as it activates the vitamin.

- Folic acid supplements (400 mcg daily) are suggested, especially for women who drink alcohol. Several important studies have shown that folic acid can help reduce breast cancer risk, including one in which women who averaged 456 mcg folic acid daily had a 44 percent lower risk of invasive breast cancer than women who took only 160 mcg folic acid.

- Green tea extract contains epigallocatechin-3-gallate (EGCG), which has been shown to inhibit breast cancer cell activity. The suggested dosage is 300 to 400 mg of standardized green tea extract daily. As a possible preventive against breast cancer, drink 2 to 4 cups of green tea daily.

- Melatonin also may inhibit the growth of certain breast cancer cells, and it has even been shown to complement the effects of some chemotherapy drugs. If you want to make melatonin part of your breast cancer prevention/treatment plan, you should talk to your healthcare provider about the most appropriate dose for your unique needs. A dose of 0.1 to 0.3 mg is the typical starting point for sleep problems, another use for melatonin, and may be used as a guide.

- Vitamin D can be an effective way to prevent breast cancer, according to researchers from the Moores Cancer Center at the University of California, San Diego. Most people are vitamin D deficient, so if you are a woman who wants to help prevent breast cancer and also boost your body's level of essential vitamin D, a supplement should be part of your daily routine. A typical dose is at least 1,000 to 2,000 IU daily. If you undergo a vitamin D test that shows you to be deficient in vitamin D, your doctor may recommend you take a higher dose for a few months until you reach a healthy level.

When to See a Doctor

Arrange to see your doctor as soon as possible if you discover a lump or you experience any of the symptoms associated with breast cancer.

COLDS/FLU

Kids catch colds. It's just a fact of life. Another fact is that one of the main reasons parents give their children nutritional and herbal supplements is to help both prevent and treat colds and flu. The best defense you and your child have against falling victim to a cold or flu virus is to strengthen the immune system. And it's a tough fight: Children younger than six years tend to have about seven colds per year, as their immune systems are still developing. Fortunately, the number of cold and flu episodes tend to decline as children get older and enter adulthood, with adults averaging one to two colds per year.

Causes and Symptoms

You and your family are exposed to more than 200 different viruses associated with the common cold and the flu, but the symptoms they cause are the same: sneezing, sore throat, nasal congestion, runny nose, coughing, headache, watery or burning eyes, and ear congestion or infection. If the flu grabs hold of you or your children, additional symptoms will likely include fever and muscle and joint aches and pains.

The viruses typically infect the cells in the nasal passages and throat, which is why the first symptom is usually a sore throat. As the virus multiplies in the body, the mucous membranes in the respiratory tract become inflamed, which makes breathing difficult. During these first few days of a cold the nasal secretions are usually watery. This is when you are most contagious and can easily transmit the virus in droplets from sneezing and coughing. When the nasal discharge turns thick and perhaps green or yellow, this indicates the presence of dead viral particles and that you are healing.

How Supplements Can Help

- Echinacea and goldenseal are the cold fighter's herbal combo. The two herbs are such a hit that you can buy them together in one supplement. The suggested dose is 250 to 500 mg of echinacea and 150 to 300 mg of goldenseal three times daily for five to seven days. Children who weigh 50 pounds may take one-third of this dose; those who weigh 100 pounds may take two-thirds the adult dose.

- Garlic is effective both in preventing and treating colds. Look for aged, standardized garlic products. The suggested dose is 600 to 1,200 mg daily in divided doses of aged garlic extract; 200 mg of freeze-dried garlic, two tablets three times daily, standardized to 1.3 percent alliin or 0.6 percent allicin. Another option is 4 mL of fluid extract daily. Children who weigh 50 pounds can take one-third the dose, while those who weigh 100 pounds can take two-thirds the dose.

- NAC can help thin and loosen mucus and relieve flu-like symptoms. A suggested dose is 600 mg three times daily. Children ages six to 12 may take one-quarter to one-half the adult dose; children older than 12 may take one-half to the complete adult dose.

- Vitamin D, not vitamin C, may be just what the doctor ordered to help prevent colds and flu. New research indicates that vitamin D is an effective cold fighter. Adults need to take at least 800 to 1,000 IU daily, while children can safely take one-quarter to one-half that amount.

• Zinc lozenges can relieve symptoms of sore throat and reduce the duration of cold symptoms, especially if you begin taking zinc within 24 hours after the appearance of cold symptoms. Zinc lozenges usually contain a 3.3 mg of elemental zinc. Adults can take one lozenge every two to four hours, not to exceed 12 lozenges daily. Children can take one-quarter to one-half the adult dose.

When to See a Doctor

If your symptoms do not improve after one week or if you experience a very high fever, shortness of breath, chest pains, or a headache along with a stiff neck, contact your physician immediately.

COLIC

If your infant cries about the same time each day (usually late afternoon or evening, but any time will do!) and nothing you do seems to offer any comfort, then your infant may have colic. The official criteria for colic is crying by an infant for more than three hours a day, three days a week for more than three weeks in an otherwise well-fed, healthy baby.

Colic can be distressing for your baby, you, and your family. It affects as many as 25 percent of babies and usually starts a few weeks after birth. The good news is that many parents see an improvement or complete disappearance of colic by three months. Some babies, however, experience symptoms for months longer, although colic ends by nine months in 90 percent of cases.

Causes and Symptoms

Experts wish they did know the cause of colic so they could perhaps offer upset and tired parents some quick cures. But they do not, so in the meantime the best we can do is relieve symptoms of colic, which include:

- Predictable crying spells that usually begin suddenly and for no apparent reason. Infants often have a bowel movement or pass gas near the end of their crying episode.

- Intense or inconsolable crying. The crying can be high pitched and cause your baby's face to become flushed.

- Changes in posture, including curled legs, clenched fists, and rigid abdominal muscles are common during episodes of colic.

How Supplements Can Help

Colic typically goes away on its own by age three months. Until then, however, you would appreciate some relief for both your baby and yourself!

- Chamomile tea has been a traditional treatment for colic for centuries. Give your infant an ounce of cooled chamomile tea in an eyedropper up to four times daily.

- Ginger tea can provide some symptom relief. Provide an ounce of cooled ginger tea in an eyedropper up to four times a day.

- Peppermint tea also can be soothing. Give your infant an ounce of cooled peppermint tea in an eye dropper up to four times a day.

- Probiotics have been shown to be helpful in some infants. Mix the contents of one probiotic capsule (about 2 billion CFUs) that contains at least five different beneficial species in formula or water. Add just enough liquid to make a slurry. Place the slurry in the nipple of a bottle, enlarge the hole, and have your baby suckle the slurry. Provide this slurry at each feeding.

When to See a Doctor

If your colicky baby does not have a healthy sucking reflex, seems uncomfortable when handled, vomits and/or loses weight, or has diarrhea or blood in the stool, call your doctor, as there could be something else going on with your child.

CONSTIPATION

Believe it or not, for a long time experts could not agree on the definition of constipation, and in fact there is still some controversy. Constipation is characterized by infrequent bowel movements, passing hard stools, and/or straining during bowel movements. The debate is around how many bowel movements a person should have each day in order to stay healthy. One to three per day used to be considered normal; today, "regular" or "normal" can mean anything from two or three bowel movements per day to one every three days.

Causes and Symptoms

Constipation can be caused by a wide variety of factors. They include:

- Dehydration
- Insufficient amount of fiber in the diet
- Ignoring the urge to have a bowel movement
- Lack of physical activity (especially in older adults or people who are ill and/or bedridden)
- Irritable bowel syndrome
- Illness
- Frequent use or abuse of laxatives

- Changes in your routine or lifestyle, such as travel
- Pregnancy (more than 50 percent of pregnant women experience constipation)
- Use of certain medications, including diuretics, high blood pressure medication, antidepressants, and pain medications
- Hormone imbalance
- Loss of fluids through vomiting or diarrhea
- Specific diseases such as diabetes, thyroid disease, Parkinson's disease, stroke
- Intestinal obstruction or diverticulosis
- Hemorrhoids
- Spinal cord injuries

Among young children, the most common causes of constipation are being afraid or unwilling to use the toilet, insufficient fiber in the diet, or a change in schedule. Drinking too much cow's milk can also cause constipation.

Symptoms of constipation can include abdominal pain, bloating, and feelings of intestinal gas that you may or may not be able to pass. Headache is also not uncommon.

How Supplements Can Help

If you can make some specific lifestyle changes for you or your child, such as adding more fiber-rich foods, reducing milk intake, and adding physical activity, constipation may be relieved. Here are some supplements that can help as well.

- Dandelion is a mild laxative that stimulates the bowel and relieves discomfort in the intestinal tract. We suggest you take dandelion along with probiotics, because dandelion contains inulin, a substance that promotes the growth of beneficial bacteria. A suggested dose is 500 mg one to three times daily of powdered root extract or 100 to 150 drops three times daily of root tincture in 45 percent alcohol. Children who weigh 50 pounds can take one-third the adult dose; at 100 pounds, two-thirds the adult dose may be taken.

• Licorice tea can soothe the intestinal tract and help relieve constipation. Adults can take licorice tea three to four times daily for three to four days; children can drink 1 to 2 cups of licorice tea daily for three to four days.

• Magnesium levels are often low in people who have constipation. You can supplement with 200 to 400 mg magnesium citrate for adults, and one-quarter to one-half this dose for children six years and older. Magnesium works in two ways: It relaxes the muscles in the intestines, and it attracts water, which softens the stool and thus helps it to pass.

• Probiotics can help break down food and keep the intestinal tract healthy. Take a probiotic supplement that contains acidophilus and several other lactobacillus and bifidobacterium species. Begin with 16 billion CFUs per meal for two to three days. As your symptoms disappear, reduce the dose to 10 billion CFUs per meal for two days, then 5 billion CFUs per meal until your symptoms are gone. Children can take one-quarter to one-half the adult dose. Probiotics can also be taken daily as a way to prevent constipation: 2 to 4 billion CFUs daily for adults and one-quarter to one-half this dose for children is suggested.

• Psyllium is a great source of fiber that can be taken as a supplement to relieve constipation. When psyllium combines with water, it swells and produces more bulk, which prompts the intestines to contract and helps move stool through the digestive tract. A typical amount of psyllium for adults is one teaspoon of the husks in water, followed by another glass of water. Children who weigh 50 pounds can take one-third the adult dose, while those weighing 100 pounds can take two-thirds the dose.

When to See a Doctor

If constipation is accompanied by fever and pain in the lower abdomen, and your stools are thin or loose when they finally are released, you may have diverticulitis. See your doctor as soon as possible. You should also contact your healthcare provider if you see blood in your stool. If constipation has lasted for a week or longer, you may have fecal impaction, a condition in which the stool has hardened in the intestinal tract. This is common among the elderly and people who are confined to bed or who are disabled. An enema may provide relief, but you may need to have a medical professional perform one if you are unable to.

DEPRESSION

Feeling down or blue once in a while is a normal part of life. But when feelings of despair and hopelessness stick around, it may be depression. Depression is the number one mental health problem in the United States, and also an equal-opportunity one: It can affect toddlers all the way to the elderly. It is estimated that 2 percent of preteen school-age children and 3 to 5 percent of teenagers have clinical depression, while the lifetime risk among women is 10 to 25 percent and among men, 5 to 12 percent. The incidence of depression is higher in the elderly.

The two main types of depression are dysthmic disorder and major clinical depression (major depressive disorder). Both types can affect children as well as adults.

- Dysthymic disorder is a type of less severe depression, but it lasts longer. You may have brief periods when your mood is normal, but then return to your mild to moderately depressed feelings. Individuals who have this disorder have symptoms of chronic depression for more than a year, with an average of three years. (See "Symptoms of Major Clinical Depression" below.) Most children who have dysthymic disorder later develop major clinical depression.

• Major depressive disorder is more severe than dysthymic disorder but lasts for an average of 32 weeks.

Another type of depression is postpartum depression, which is believed to be caused, at least in part, by an imbalance in hormones levels that occurs after childbirth. Women who experience postpartum depression typically regain their equilibrium within several weeks to months after delivery, once their hormone levels are restored.

Depression among the elderly is often missed and not treated because they may deny they are feeling overwhelmingly sad or be ashamed of their feelings. Older adults show the same symptoms of depression already mentioned, but they may also express other signals, such as pacing, showing little or no interest in personal care, an increase in aches and pains, and fretting excessively about their health, their money, or the state of the world. It is important to know that anyone who is depressed can get help, regardless of age.

Causes and Symptoms

Research suggests that depression is associated with the suppression of the growth of new brain cells, stress, and changes in hormone levels. The theory is that among people who are depressed, the brain stops making new nerve cells. Stress can cause the body to release excessive amount of certain hormones to the brain, where they suppress the generation of new nerve cells. When hormone levels are restored and stress is relieved, depression can go away.

Experts have devised a list of typical symptoms to help them (and you) identify the symptoms of major depression (see below). Among children and adolescents, there are some developmental variations that can serve as signals to parents.

SYMPTOMS OF MAJOR DEPRESSION (MAJOR DEPRESSIVE DISORDER)

- Feelings of helplessness and hopelessness
- Loss of interest in daily activities, including former hobbies, social activities, and sex
- Changes in appetite or weight
- Sleep problems, either insomnia or oversleeping
- Irritability or restlessness
- Lack of energy, feeling fatigued and physically drained
- Strong feelings of guilt or worthlessness
- Difficulty concentrating, making decisions, or remembering things
- Thoughts of death, suicide ideation and/or attempts

For example, children ages six to 12 may also display difficulties with school, make negative statements, complain a lot, show eating disturbances, and appear bored or apathetic. Among older children (ages 12 to 18), additional symptoms to look for include acting out sexually, social isolation, drug and/or alcohol use, and rage.

How Supplements Can Help

An important study published in January 2010 in the *Journal of the American Medical Association* reported that antidepressants are little better than a placebo for people who have mild to moderate depression. This finding is fuel for those who want to turn to natural supplements to treat depression. Here are some of the options.

- A high-potency B-complex is suggested, along with some extra B vitamins until your symptoms are resolved. The extra B vitamins to take include 300 to

500 mcg vitamin B_{12} twice daily; 800 mcg folic acid once daily; and 50 mg vitamin B_6 twice daily for two weeks, then once daily.

- Omega-3 fatty acids have been shown to improve symptoms of major depression in adults, especially when taken along with conventional treatment to which patients have not responded. Research also indicates that omega-3 fatty acids are safe for pregnant women who are suffering from depression. Although there is no standard dose of omega-3 fatty acids for treatment of depression, many studies have shown 1 gram of the omega-3 EPA (eicosapentoaenoic acid) daily to be effective.

- SAM-e has been shown to be equal or superior to prescription antidepressants in more than 100 studies, and without the side effects. The suggested starting dose for adults is 400 mg daily, which can be gradually increased up to 1,600 mg daily as needed. Talk to your doctor before giving SAM-e to your child.

- St. John's wort gradually alters brain chemistry similar to the way conventional antidepressants do. A starting dose of St. John's wort is typically 300 mg daily of standardized extract containing 0.3 percent hypericin. Increase the daily dose by 300 mg after two weeks, and then by another 300 mg after another two weeks. The same amount of St. John's wort has been found to be both safe and effective in children younger than 12. Talk to your healthcare professional before taking St. John's wort if you have high blood pressure.

When to See a Doctor

Generally it is best to have a professional evaluation before you treat yourself or your children for depression. Consult a physician if your child or an elderly parent shows indications of or mentions suicide, or their daily activities are significantly impaired because of their depression.

DIABETES

Diabetes is a chronic condition in which the body is unable to either produce or properly utilize insulin. Approximately 23.6 million people in the United States have diabetes, which represents 7.8 percent of the population. The two main types of diabetes are type 1 and type 2. Type 1 diabetes, which used to be called juvenile-onset diabetes, can first appear anytime from infancy (although this is rare) up through early adulthood. The chances of developing type 1 diabetes peaks in early puberty and declines thereafter. About 10 percent of people who have diabetes have type 1.

Type 2 diabetes traditionally has appeared a bit later in life, usually around age 40. In recent years, however, a growing number of younger people have been diagnosed with type 2 diabetes. The incidence of type 2 diabetes among adolescents has increased tenfold over the last decade. This phenomenon has been associated with the high number of young people who are overweight or obese, as type 2 diabetes is closely associated with excess weight. About 85 to 90 percent of people who have diabetes have type 2.

Basically, the difference between the two types of diabetes is that in type 1 diabetes, the pancreas does not produce the insulin the body needs in order to move glucose into the cells. In type 2 diabetes, the pancreas does produce insulin, but the body's cells are resistant to its effects, so the insulin can't do its job.

Although the causes of these two different types of diabetes are not the same, the outcome basically is: the cells do not get enough fuel (glucose) and the glucose accumulates in the bloodstream and rises to unhealthy levels, which can then lead to a variety of symptoms and complications, including

CLINICIANS MAKE A DIAGNOSIS OF DIABETES IF ANY OF THE FOLLOWING ARE TRUE:

- Your blood glucose level is greater than or equal to 200 mg/dL two hours after you have ingested 75 grams of glucose
- Your fasting blood glucose is greater than or equal to 126 mg/dL
- Your blood glucose is 200 mg/dL and you have symptoms of diabetes (see below)

damage to the kidneys, eyes, nervous system, heart, skin, and blood vessels.

Causes and Symptoms

For type 1 diabetes, experts do not know exactly why the pancreas does not produce insulin as it was designed to do. They do know, however, that the body's immune system mistakenly destroys the cells (islet) in the pancreas that produce insulin. Once the islet cells are destroyed, the pancreas is unable to produce insulin. This autoimmune response by the body could be the result of an inherited tendency as well as environmental factors. The end result is that people who have type 1 diabetes must take insulin every day.

Type 2 diabetes develops when the body becomes resistant to insulin or when the pancreas stops producing enough of the hormone. Although the exact reason why this happens is not known, being overweight and inactivity are important risk factors. We know, for example, that the more fatty tissue you have the more resistant your cells are to insulin, and that physical activity helps control weight, allows cells to consume glucose as energy, and makes them more sensitive to insulin.

Symptoms of both types of diabetes include frequent hunger, excessive thirst, frequent urination, fatigue, weakness, weight loss, dehydration, and in women, persistent vaginal infections.

How Supplements Can Help

- Cinnamon can help control blood glucose levels and also lower triglyceride and cholesterol levels. A suggested dose is 125 mg of extract standardized to 0.95 percent trimeric and tetrameric A-type polymers (active ingredients in cinnamon) three times daily. An alternative is to use 3 to 6 g powdered whole cinnamon daily. Children who weigh 50 pounds can take one-third the adult dose; at 100 pounds, they can take two-thirds the dose.

- Coenzyme Q_{10} may help control blood sugar levels, high cholesterol, and high blood pressure in people with type 2 diabetes. A suggested dose is 200 mg twice daily. Consult your doctor before giving CoQ_{10} to your child.

- Ginseng can improve glucose and insulin control. A suggested dose is 200 mg of standardized extract at 4 percent ginsenosides, an active ingredient. Children who weigh 50 pounds can take one-third the adult dose; those weighing 100 pounds can take a two-thirds dose.

- Magnesium levels are typically low in people who have type 2 diabetes. Some studies indicate that taking magnesium supplements may help control blood sugar and insulin sensitivity. A suggested dose is 160 mg three times daily. Children may take one-quarter to one-half the adult dose.

- Pycnogenol has been shown to lower blood sugar levels and relieve diabetic retinopathy, a complication of diabetes in which leaking blood vessels in the eyes can cause vision loss. The suggested dose of pycnogenol is 100 to 200 mg daily. Children younger than six years should not take pycnogenol. The dose for children who weigh 50 pounds is one-third the adult dose; for children weighing 100 pounds, the dose is two-thirds.

When to See a Doctor

Contact your doctor if you are having difficulty regulating your glucose levels, if you are experiencing frequent episodes of hypoglycemia (low blood sugar), or if you develop new symptoms.

DIARRHEA

If we can say one good thing about diarrhea, it would be that it allows the body to eliminate substances that are irritating it, including allergens, medications, bacteria, and viruses. The not-so-great news is that it can make you feel pretty miserable and stressed until the episode has been resolved. For everyone, but especially for children and the elderly, chronic diarrhea or diarrhea that lasts for days and days can cause dehydration.

When you or a family member has diarrhea, the food and fluids that you ingest pass too rapidly or in too large an amount, or both, through your colon. The result is a watery bowel movement. At the same time, the body fails to sufficiently absorb the nutrients from the food. If the lining of the colon is inflamed or diseased, it will be less able to absorb fluids, and dehydration may occur.

Causes and Symptoms

Diarrhea is often caused by viruses, including the Norwalk virus, viral hepatitis, cytomegalovirus, and the herpes simplex virus. Among children, the most common cause of acute diarrhea is the rotavirus. Bacteria and parasites can also cause diarrhea, including those that may be lurking in spoiled or improperly stored food (food poisoning), or what is commonly referred to as traveler's diarrhea. The warning "don't drink the water" when traveling to certain foreign countries is given for this very reason. Less often, diarrhea can be caused by certain medications (e.g., antibiotics), lactose, fructose (a common cause of diarrhea in children), artificial sweeteners, and digestive disorders such as Crohn's disease, ulcerative colitis, and irritable bowel syndrome.

Symptoms of diarrhea include watery stools, abdominal cramps or pain, fever, bloating, and blood in the stool. Diarrhea caused by an infection may be accompanied by nausea and vomiting.

How Supplements Can Help

- Garlic tea may sound a bit unappetizing, but if you think of it as garlic soup, doesn't it suddenly sound more appetizing? Garlic can kill bacteria and viruses, so this broth can be helpful. Bake six unpeeled garlic cloves in the oven for ten minutes at 350°F, then boil the cloves in 30 ounces of water for 8 minutes. Strain and drink 10 ounces of the broth every three hours until your symptoms disappear. You may be able to get your child to try this if you put some cooked noodles into the broth and make it a "soup." Or you can go the supplement route and take three 500 mg capsules of garlic daily.

- Ginger can ease symptoms of diarrhea and is a flavor that can appeal to children. Mix one teaspoon of ginger juice in 4 ounces of boiling water and drink three to four times a day. A variation is to mix ½ teaspoon each of ginger juice and lemon juice, and ¼ teaspoon pepper powder in 4 ounces of boiling water. Drink twice daily. Children can be treated using one-third to two-thirds of the adult dose, based on their body weight.

- Peppermint has antispasmodic properties, so several cups of peppermint tea can relieve intestinal cramping. A typical adult dose is 3 cups of tea daily: Steep 1 to 2 teaspoons of dried peppermint leaf in 1 cup of hot water for 10 minutes. Children tend to like the peppermint tea, but use one-third to two-thirds of the adult dose, based on body weight.

- Probiotics help restore balance to the intestinal tract and clear out the organisms that are causing the diarrhea. Begin with a probiotic supplement that contains at least three different species and take 16 billion CFUs per meal for five days or until your symptoms disappear completely. Then take 2 to 3 billion CFUs daily to help support your healed intestinal tract. Children can take one-quarter to one-half the adult dose. Probiotics can also be taken daily as a way to prevent diarrhea: 2 to 4 billion CFUs daily for adults and one-quarter to one-half this dose for children is suggested.

When to See a Doctor

If you are an adult and your diarrhea persists for more than three days, if you become dehydrated or have severe abdominal or rectal pain, or if you have bloody stools or a temperature of more than 102°F, you should see your doctor. In children, diarrhea can quickly result in dehydration. If your child's diarrhea has not improved within 24 hours or if your baby cries without tears, has a dry mouth, has bloody or black stools, is unusually sleepy, has a fever greater than 102°F, or hasn't had a wet diaper in more than three hours, contact your physician.

EAR INFECTIONS

Few children make it through childhood without experiencing at least one middle ear infection. In fact, 75 percent of children have had at least one ear infection (also known as otitis media) by age three, according to the National Institute on Deafness and Other Communication Disorders. Most children stop having ear infections by age five.

Ear infections also occur in adults, but much less often. Children are more susceptible to ear infections because the Eustachian tube, which connects the nasal cavity and the inner ear, is straighter, shorter, and more horizontal in children than in adults. This gives bacteria a free ride to the inner ear, where they can take hold and cause infection.

Causes and Symptoms

The two most common types of ear infection are middle ear infections and swimmer's ear. Middle ear infections are caused by bacteria that attack the middle ear. These infections are often a complication of the common cold or other upper respiratory infections, such as infection of the adenoids, tonsils, or sinuses. Symptoms include pain and swelling behind the eardrum, chills, sore throat, muffled hearing, and a feeling of fullness in the affected ear.

Swimmer's ear, also called otitis externa, is characterized by an itchy or blocked feeling in the ear, tenderness or pain when moving your head, temporary hearing loss, and a yellow or watery discharge from the ear. More adults than children get swimmer's ear. Although you don't need to be a swimmer to develop this type of ear infection, getting polluted or chlorinated water in your ears is the main cause.

How Supplements Can Help

Most ear infections clear up on their own within a few days, but in the meantime, your child (or you) can be very uncomfortable. Here are some natural supplements that can help.

- Echinacea tincture is helpful for some children who have recurrent middle ear infections. The suggested dose is 1 to 2 mL (depending on the child's age; start at the lowest dose) of echinacea tincture taken three times daily. Begin supplementation as soon as the symptoms appear and continue until a few days after they are gone.

- Garlic oil can kill the bacteria that are involved in swimmer's ear. Place a few drops of garlic oil on a cotton ball and put the cotton in your ear overnight. You can also add a few drops of St. John's wort to the cotton ball. Treatment for children and adults is the same.

- Goldenseal capsules or tincture can boost the immune system and speed up recovery. The adult dose is 500 mg to 2 g of dried root in capsules three times daily, or ½ to 1 tsp of liquid extract in water three times daily. To treat your child, multiply the adult dose (start at the low end) by the child's weight, then divide by 150.

- Probiotics are recommended for your child, especially if he or she is taking antibiotics, which destroy the good bacteria along with the bad in the intestinal tract. A suggested dose is 12 to 15 billion CFUs of a probiotic supplement that contains three or more species, taken daily until the infection clears. Adults can take two to three times this dose.

When to See a Doctor

If you, your child, or other family member experiences a high fever, severe pain, or other complications along with the ear infection, seek immediate medical attention. If your infant has a fever, contact your doctor immediately, regardless of other symptoms he or she may be experiencing. If ear infections are a chronic problem, talk to your doctor, as they may be caused by a food allergy, with dairy products and wheat being the most common culprits.

ECZEMA

Eczema, also known as atopic dermatitis, is a chronic skin condition that affects more than 15 million people in the United States. It is most often seen in infants and young children, affecting between 10 and 20 percent of all infants. Sixty-five percent of patients develop symptoms of eczema before their first birthday, and 90 percent of them have symptoms before the age of five. Fortunately, eczema usually disappears by age three. This condition is much less common among adults, but for them the rash is usually chronic or recurring and limited to the inner elbow or behind the knee. Eczema appears to frequently affect people who have family members with asthma, hay fever, or eczema as well. In fact, 75 percent of children with eczema go on to develop hay fever or asthma.

Causes and Symptoms

The exact cause of eczema is not known, but experts generally agree that it is associated with an overactive response by the body's immune system to various triggers. For example, some people experience a flare-up of the rash when they come into contact with certain soaps, fabrics, or animal dander. Upper respiratory infections or colds, which are common among infants and young children, may also be triggers.

Among infants and children, the rash that is associated with eczema most often appears on the cheeks, knees, and elbows and is red, itchy, and scaly. The skin can become thick and leathery from chronic irritation and scratching. Sometimes eczema oozes or it can look dry. The symptoms can get worse when it is dry, the temperature changes, the rash is exposed to water, and/or the patient experiences stress. Among adults with eczema, stress appears to be an exacerbating factor.

How Supplements Can Help

• Licorice gel has proven superior to placebo in the treatment of eczema. After two weeks, use of both 1 percent and 2 percent licorice gels have been more effective at relieving symptoms of redness, swelling, and itching than placebo, but the 2 percent gel works better than the 1 percent.

• Probiotics appear to help both prevent and treat eczema in children. A large, two-year study of infants and their mothers found that those who received a probiotic supplement for six months were significantly more likely to avoid developing eczema than those who took a placebo. Studies have also indicated that certain probiotic strains may help treat infants and children who already have eczema. Those strains include *Lactobacillus G, L. reuteri, L. rhamnosus, L. fermentum VRI-033 PCC,* and *Bifidobacteria lactis.* The following is the suggested adult dose; children can be given one-quarter to one-half this amount. Begin with 16.5 billion CFUs of a multi-strain probiotic taken with meals for five days, followed by 11 billion CFUs per meal for another five days, and then 5.5 billion CFUs per meal until the symptoms disappear or are under control.

• Quercetin has anti-inflammatory properties and may also strengthen connective tissue and reduce symptoms of an allergic reaction. The adult dose is 50 to 250 mg two to three times daily. Consult your doctor before giving quercetin to infants. Children ages two years and older can take one-quarter to one-half the adult dose.

• St. John's wort applied as a topical cream has shown promise. The cream can be applied to the affected areas as often as instructed on the product for both adults and children. Look for a cream that contains 1.5 percent hyperforin.

- Vitamin E can be taken orally and applied to the affected skin. An adult dose of vitamin E is 400 IU daily for two weeks, then add 400 IU in the evening for two, and finally add yet another 400 IU in the middle of the day, for a total of 1,200 IU daily. Continue until symptoms disappear. Consult your doctor before giving vitamin E to infants. Dosing for children ages two years and older may be one-quarter to one-half the adult dose. To use vitamin E on the skin, you can pierce a vitamin E capsule and squeeze out the oil onto the skin. Apply to the affected areas once or twice daily.

When to See a Doctor

If your or your child's symptoms have not improved after two weeks of self-treatment, you may need a prescription. You may also consult a physician if the eczema begins to ooze, has an odor, begins to crust over, or shows signs of infection, such as redness, swelling, or pus.

ERECTILE DYSFUNCTION

Erectile dysfunction (ED) is the inability to attain and maintain an erection that is sufficient for satisfactory sexual activity. Approximately 30 million men in the United States experience ED, and the prevalence increases with age. For example, while about 5 percent of men have ED at age 40, up to 50 percent or higher experience it at age 65 and older. Although ED used to be a topic that people—especially men—didn't talk about, the pendulum has certainly swung the other way, and now there are commercials and stories about ED on television, radio, and other media. This is good news, because it encourages more and more men to seek help.

Causes and Symptoms

In about 90 percent of cases, erectile dysfunction is the result of a physical or medical problem. Because adequate blood flow to the penis is essential for an erection to occur, any factor or health condition that impedes that flow can cause ED. Therefore, diabetes, high blood pressure, high cholesterol, cardiovascular disease, stroke, and renal failure, as well as Parkinson's disease, spinal cord injuries, and multiple sclerosis all may cause ED.

Some drugs also may cause ED, including antidepressants, most antihypertensive drugs, calcium channel blockers, ACE inhibitors, cimetidine (for duodenal ulcers), and finasteride (for prostate enlargement and baldness). If you are currently taking any of these drugs and are also experiencing ED, you should talk to your doctor about changing your medication.

In about 10 percent of cases, psychological problems cause ED. These problems may include obsessive-compulsive personality disorder, depression, psychotic disorders, an intense fear of failure, and a stressful relationship with the sex partner.

How Supplements Can Help

Although there are several prescription drugs on the market that have proved quite successful in treating ED, they are not without side effects, and they also can be costly. Several natural supplements may provide just the help you need.

• The amino acid arginine enhances the effects of nitric oxide, which is the same effect that Viagra and other similar ED medications have on the body. The suggested dosage is 3,000 mg daily. The drawback is that it does not work like ED drugs because you need to take it for several weeks before you will notice any response. Do not take arginine if you have genital herpes.

- Ginkgo biloba is known for its ability to improve circulation, and in this case it enhances blood flow to the penis. Ginkgo is for the patient man: It may take from two to six months to notice significant results. The suggested daily dose is 60 mg.

- Ginseng, both American and Asian, have been shown in several studies to be helpful in treating erectile dysfunction. Like arginine, ginseng is believed to increase nitric oxide synthesis, which increases blood flow. A suggested dose is 500 mg one to three times daily of a standardized ginseng powder containing 5 percent ginsenosides (the active ingredients). If you select a ginseng supplement that contains 18 percent ginsenoside, take 150 mg one to three times daily.

- Zinc can be helpful, especially in men who have low levels of this mineral associated with long-term use of diuretics, diabetes, digestive disorders, and certain liver and kidney diseases. A suggested dose is 30 mg daily, along with 400 IU vitamin E, to help support hormone production.

When to See a Doctor

If all of your efforts have not been successful, you may have an undetected medical condition. It may be time to see a urologist to explore other options.

GOUT

Gout is a common type of arthritis that often affects the big toe, resulting in a condition known as "gouty big toe" or "gouty arthritis." Few people are aware, however, that gout can also affect the ears, heel of the hand, small hand joints, ankles, knees, elbows, and wrists. Of course, if you are among the estimated 3 million adults who have gout, you may already know that.

Seventy-five to 90 percent of people who develop gout are male, and most of them first get the condition after age 40. Most of the women who get gout develop it postmenopause. Children rarely get this form of arthritis.

Causes and Symptoms

People who have gout do not have enough of a digestive enzyme called uricase, which is necessary to break down and excrete uric acid, a byproduct of the digestion of certain foods. The result is that the uric acid accumulates and forms crystals, which then causes symptoms of inflammation, swelling, and intense pain. These symptoms usually come on suddenly and can last from a few hours to several days. If the condition is not controlled, excessive excretion of uric acid in the urine can lead to the development of kidney stones, kidney disease, and even kidney failure.

Certain foods and beverages can cause uric acid levels to rise in the blood and lead to the formation of crystals. To help prevent gout, avoid alcohol, anchovies, asparagus, coffee, legumes, meat, mushrooms, shellfish, and soft drinks. These foods and beverages contain purines, substances that contribute to the development of gout. Other causes of gout include stress; a deficiency of vitamins A, B_5, and E; chemotherapy; and diseases such as psoriasis and leukemia.

How Supplements Can Help

- The amino acids glutamine and methionine can help detoxify the purines. The suggested doses are 500 mg of glutamine four times daily and 250 mg methionine twice daily, both on an empty stomach. Do not give amino acid supplements to children.

- B-complex supplements plus an extra amount of vitamin B_5 can help the body convert uric acid into harmless compounds. The suggested dose is one to three 50-mg B-complex tablets daily, plus 500 mg vitamin

B_5, all in divided doses. Children can take one-quarter to one-half the adult dose.

- Devil's claw can reduce uric acid levels. Take 400 mg of dried extract three times daily both as a preventive measure and treatment. Children weighing 50 pounds may be given one-third the adult dose; at 100 pounds, they can take two-thirds the dose.

- Magnesium is an effective antispasmodic and can relieve the pain of gout. The suggested dose is 400 mg magnesium citrate three times daily. Children can be given one-quarter to one-half the adult dose.

- Quercetin inhibits the production of uric acid in a way similar to drugs prescribed to treat this disease. The suggested dose is 1,000 mg along with 1,000 to 1,500 mg of the enzyme bromelain (which enhances absorption) two to three times daily.

When to See a Doctor

Consult your doctor if you do not experience relief from your symptoms after a week or two and/or if your affected joint(s) become swollen, warm, and flushed.

HEARTBURN/GERD

Heartburn, indigestion, dyspepsia—call it what you will, it's that burning feeling in your chest and sour, awful taste in your mouth that occurs after eating. It can last for just a few minutes or for up to several hours. Heartburn is the symptom you feel when acid rises up and out of the stomach into your throat. More than 60 million adults in America suffer from heartburn at least once a month, and about 25 million have the experience on a daily basis. Heartburn tends to be more common among the elderly and pregnant women.

The term "heartburn" is sometimes used interchangeably with "acid reflux." Heartburn is often thought of as an adult condition, but infants, young children, and adolescents are no strangers to heartburn. GERD, or gastroesophageal reflux disease, a chronic or severe form of acid reflux, affects up to 50 percent of infants less than three months old. Spitting up is a common sign of GERD, but it is believed that many infants also have heartburn. It is also estimated that 2 percent of children ages three to nine and 5 percent of those ages 10 to 17 experience heartburn. One estimate is that 19 million Americans suffer from GERD.

Causes and Symptoms

Because heartburn and GERD are related, we can explain them together. Heartburn is the main symptom of GERD, in which the liquid contents of the stomach regurgitate (reflux) into the esophagus. Symptoms of heartburn include:

- a burning feeling in the chest just behind the breastbone that develops after eating
- A hot, sour, acidic, or salty-tasting fluid at the back of the throat
- Trouble swallowing
- A feeling like food is stuck in the middle of your chest or throat
- Chest pain, especially after you eat, bend over, or lie down
- Chronic cough, sore throat, or chronic hoarseness

Regurgitation occurs when the sphincter (a ring of muscle at the bottom of the esophagus) malfunctions and relaxes when you are not swallowing. This allows liquids from the stomach to rise up out of the stomach into the esophagus. These liquids burn because they contain hydrochloric acid and an enzyme called pepsin, which help digest your food. The regurgitated fluids also may contain bile, which can enter the stomach from the small intestine.

In infants and young children, heartburn is usually a sign
of GERD, and it is usually caused by an immature digestive
tract. In older children, risks for heartburn and GERD include
being overweight, eating certain foods (e.g., fatty foods, spicy
foods, carbonated beverages), eating large portions, and exposure to secondhand smoke. Heartburn in adults can be caused
by the same factors, as well as smoking, lying down immediately after eating, drinking alcohol or coffee, pregnancy, use
of aspirin or ibuprofen, and a stomach abnormality called hiatal hernia, in which the upper part of the stomach and the
lower esophagus slide up into the chest through an opening
call the hiatus.

Among children who have reflux disease, the most common symptom is recurrent abdominal pain that is worse
around the upper part of the abdomen, followed by heartburn. Children who had a history of recurrent vomiting during infancy are more likely to develop heartburn and GERD
later in life.

How Supplements Can Help

- Aloe vera juice can soothe an irritated esophagus. A
  suggested dose for adults is 2 ounces of aloe vera juice
  taken about 20 minutes before each meal. Pregnant
  women should not use aloe vera juice, and it generally
  is not recommended for children.

- Licorice promotes mucus secretion in the stomach and
  can help resolve too much stomach acid. Look for deglycyrrhizinated licorice (DGL), the form of the herb
  that has had the glycyrrhizin component removed, as
  it can cause high blood pressure. A suggested dose is
  380 mg (this equals about two wafers) taken three or
  four times daily between meals. For children who
  weigh 50 pounds, one-third of the adult dose is suggested; for children weighing 100 pounds, the dose
  can be two-thirds of the adult dose.

- MSM can relieve symptoms of heartburn. Begin with 1 level teaspoon of MSM powder (5 grams) dissolved in water. Take this two to three times daily. You can increase the dose by 1 teaspoon per day if symptoms are not relieved with the lower dose. This dose is also safe for children, although you will probably have to mix it into a tasty beverage, as MSM has a bitter taste.

- Probiotics restore good bacteria to the gut and relieve symptoms of heartburn and GERD. A suggested adult dose is 2.5 to 5.5 billion CFUs of a probiotic supplement that contains at least four to five species. Take the supplement with each meal until symptoms are under control. Children can take one-quarter to one-half the adult dose.

- Slippery elm is known for its ability to soothe an irritated esophagus, throat, and stomach. A suggested adult dose is two to three tablets or capsules each containing 400 to 500 mg three times daily. An alternative is slippery elm tea prepared by steeping 1 to 2 grams of slippery elm bark in 8 oz of boiled water for 10 minutes. For best results, drink 3 to 4 cups of tea daily. Children weighing 50 pounds can take one-third the oral supplement dose or drink 1 cup daily (several ounces each dose); those who weigh 100 pounds can take two-thirds the adult oral supplement dose or drink 2 cups daily. To sweeten the tea, you can add a little cinnamon or ginger, both of which offer some soothing qualities for heartburn themselves.

When to See a Doctor

Heartburn and especially a hiatal hernia can cause chest pain, which can easily be confused with a heart attack. That's why it is so important to get an evaluation and a diagnosis from your doctor if you experience unexplained chest pain. When infants or children experience chronic heartburn or GERD, it is best to see a physician to make sure there is no damage to the esophagus or throat and to get an accurate diagnosis.

HEMORRHOIDS

Hemorrhoids, which are also known as piles, are swollen and inflamed veins in the anus and rectum. More than 75 percent of people in the United States experience hemorrhoids at some point during their lives, although they mostly appear in individuals between the ages of 45 and 65. Hemorrhoids can occur either inside (internal) or outside (external) the anus.

Some people are surprised to learn that hemorrhoids can affect children, that is, unless your child has this condition. Fortunately, hemorrhoids in children are typically mild and of short duration, and do not require treatment.

Sometimes people confuse hemorrhoids with anal fissures. If you see spots of blood on toilet paper and have painful bowel movements, you may have an anal fissure, which is often caused by constipation. If your stools are dry and hard and you are experiencing sharp, stinging, often severe pain when having a bowel movement, chances are you have an anal fissure and not hemorrhoids, as hemorrhoids typically cause bleeding but no pain.

The best way to prevent hemorrhoids (and anal fissures) is to get adequate fiber in your diet (e.g., lots of fresh fruits and vegetables and whole grains), drink enough fluids, and participate in daily physical exercise, which promotes a healthy intestinal tract.

Causes and Symptoms

The causes of hemorrhoids are largely preventable. For example:

- Constipation: This is one of the main causes of hemorrhoids in both children and adults, because straining puts a great deal of pressure on the veins in the anus. As we noted, an insufficient amount of fiber in the diet, inadequate intake of fluids, and lack of exercise all contribute to constipation. (Also see the entry on "Constipation.")

• Pregnancy: Expectant moms often experience hemorrhoids, which are caused by a combination of hormonal changes and increased pressure imposed by the growing fetus on the veins to pump blood.

• Weakness in the veins: This condition, which is also known as chronic venous insufficiency, can result in hemorrhoids in people who are overweight or who smoke, stand or sit for long periods, or who do not get enough exercise.

• Inflammatory bowel disease: If you have Crohn's disease or ulcerative colitis, it can be an underlying cause of hemorrhoids.

• Portal hypertension: This is a type of hypertension in which there is increased pressure within the portal vein that runs from the intestines to the liver. The most common cause of portal hypertension is liver cirrhosis.

• Aging: No one avoids this one. As people age, the support structures in the area of the anus weaken, resulting in hemorrhoids in some people.

• Parents: Some children have a tendency to get hemorrhoids if their mother also had them during pregnancy. Also, children are more apt to develop hemorrhoids if both parents suffer from the condition.

If you have internal hemorrhoids, symptoms typically include painless bleeding at the end of a bowel movement. You may also experience a sensation of fullness, a feeling like you need to have a bowel movement even when there is no stool. You may have itching, acute pain, and irritation around the anus. This often happens when the hemorrhoid can be seen outside the anus or if a blood clot forms. These can be serious and should be seen by a doctor. External hemorrhoids are often felt as a lump or bulge in the anus. Although they are usually painful and itchy, they do not always cause typical symptoms.

How Supplements Can Help

- Aloe vera can be applied topically to hemorrhoids to relieve itching and burning. This is helpful for both children and adults, applied as often as needed.

- Dandelion tincture or capsules can help soften hard stools. A suggested dose is 500 mg one to three times daily of powdered root extract or 100 to 150 drops three times daily of root tincture in 45 percent alcohol. Children who weigh 50 pounds can take one-third the adult dose; at 100 pounds, two-thirds the adult dose may be taken.

- Psyllium can help keep your intestinal tract healthy and prevent constipation, a major cause of hemorrhoids. A typical amount of psyllium for adults is one teaspoon of the husks in water, followed by another glass of water. Children who weigh 50 pounds can take one-third the adult dose, while those weighing 100 pounds can take two-thirds the dose.

- Pycnogenol, both orally and topically, has recently been found to be effective in treating hemorrhoids. The suggested dose for adults is six 50-mg tablets per day for four days, then three 50-mg tablets for three days. At the same time, apply topical 0.5 percent pycnogenol cream to the affected area to relieve itching and other symptoms.

- Vitamin E oil applied on the affected area with a cotton swab several times a day can be soothing. If you can't find vitamin E oil, simply stick a pin into a vitamin E capsule and squeeze out the oil.

When to See a Doctor

It's time to see your doctor if you develop bleeding between bowel movements, you experience a moderate amount of bleeding from hemorrhoids, you are older than 40 or have a family history of colon cancer and are experiencing rectal bleeding, you have prolapsed hemorrhoids that will not go back through the anus, or you have significant pain from your hemorrhoids. If you have a large amount of bleeding from your rectum or become dizzy or weak, you should seek immediate medical assistance.

HIGH BLOOD PRESSURE

High blood pressure, also known as hypertension, is a condition in which the degree of pressure inside the blood vessels and the pressure created when the heart beats is elevated. Blood pressure values are measured in millimeters of mercury (mmHg) and are given using two numbers. For example, for the value 120 over 80 (120/80 mmHg), the 120 is the systolic pressure, or the pressure created when the heart beats, while 80 is the diastolic pressure, which is the pressure inside the blood vessels when the heart is at rest. Physicians identify a person's blood pressure status using the following guidelines:

- Normal blood pressure is less than 120/80 mmHg
- Prehypertension is systolic pressure that is between 120 and 139 or diastolic pressure between 80 and 89
- Stage 1 hypertension is systolic pressure between 140 to 159 or diastolic pressure between 90 and 99
- Stage 2 hypertension is systolic pressure greater than 160 or diastolic pressure greater than 100

About one-third of adults in the United States have high blood pressure. This is of great concern, given that high blood pressure is a major risk factor for heart disease, stroke, kidney disease, and congestive heart failure. It is also a primary or contributing cause of death for more than 326,000 Americans per year. About 25 percent of American adults have prehypertension. Women and men are about equally likely to develop high blood pressure during their lifetimes, but among people younger than 45, more men than women are affected. After age 65, it affects more women than men.

The elderly are at an increased risk for high blood pressure, because the arterial walls tend to lose elasticity with age, which causes the pressure of the blood traveling through the arteries to rise. Therefore it is especially important for older adults to have their blood pressure checked regularly and for elevated blood pressure to be treated.

Children, even infants, can have high blood pressure. According to a study published in *Pediatrics,* the prevalence of high blood pressure among children ranges from 5.4 to 19.4 percent. That's why the American Heart Association recommends that all children age three and older have their blood pressure checked each year. Early detection of high blood pressure allows you and your doctor to take steps to treat this condition, because it is a major risk factor for heart disease and stroke in adulthood.

Causes and Symptoms

In children, high blood pressure can be caused by other diseases, such as kidney or heart disease. Children who are overweight usually have higher blood pressure than children who are of normal weight. High blood pressure can also be inherited if one or both parents have hypertension, and it is more frequent and severe in blacks than in whites.

Among adults, factors that can cause and contribute to high blood pressure include smoking, being overweight or obese, a lack of physical exercise, a high-salt diet, consuming more than two alcoholic drinks per day, stress, older age, genetics, family history of high blood pressure, chronic kidney disease, and thyroid and adrenal disorders.

People who have high blood pressure typically do not experience any symptoms, which is the main reason this condition can be so dangerous, since the first indication that someone has high blood pressure may be a stroke. Someone who has very high blood pressure (160 over 100 or higher) may experience a hypertensive crisis, with symptoms that include pulsating headache that occurs behind the eyes, nausea and vomiting, and visual disturbances. This is an emergency situation that requires immediate attention.

How Supplements Can Help

- Coenzyme Q_{10} can significantly lower blood pressure. Studies in adults show that 60 to 100 mg twice daily for 12 weeks can be very effective. In younger people, you should consult your pediatrician before giving this supplement to children younger than 18 years old. Typically, children are given one-quarter to one-half the adult dose.

- Garlic can lower systolic or diastolic blood pressure, or both. Because garlic can make your blood thinner or interact with some other drugs or supplements (e.g., warfarin, aspirin, vitamin E, ginkgo), you should talk to your doctor before taking garlic for hypertension. A suggested dose for adults is 900 mg daily standardized to 0.6 percent allicin.

- Hawthorn is a traditional herb for high blood pressure, and scientific research has shown there is good reason for using this herb. A suggested dose for adults is 1,200 mg daily in divided doses. Talk to your doctor before giving your child hawthorn for high blood pressure.

- Magnesium and calcium can help lower high blood pressure if you are deficient in these essential minerals. Women should consume 1,000 to 1,200 mg of calcium daily from all sources, while men should get no more than 500 to 600 mg daily, according to Dr. Andrew Weil. Magnesium intake should be about half of the calcium.

- Omega-3 can have a modest impact on blood pressure. Although fish oil supplements usually contain both DHA and EPA, there is evidence that DHA is the one that lowers high blood pressure. To lower blood pressure, take 2 g of omega-3 supplements two to three times daily. Children may be treated with a dose that is one-third to two-thirds of this level, depending on their body weight.

When to See a Doctor

Because high blood pressure typically does not have noticeable symptoms, it is important to have regular physical exams to make sure your blood pressure is within a normal range. This is especially important if you have a family history of hypertension, if you are overweight, or if you have ever had high blood pressure. If you are already being treated for high blood pressure and you experience shortness of breath, excessive sweating, vision problems, confusion, nausea, or lightheadedness, contact your physician.

HIGH CHOLESTEROL

High cholesterol, or hypercholesterolemia for those who like big words, is defined as the presence of 240 mcg/dL (microgram of cholesterol per deciliter of blood) or greater of a fatlike substance in the bloodstream. A level between 200 and 239 mg/dL is considered borderline high cholesterol, while less than 200 mg/dL is considered normal. Cholesterol is a fat-like substance that plays both good guy and bad guy in the body. While cholesterol is necessary for many functions, including the production of certain hormones, too much cholesterol can cause health problems.

An estimated 42 million Americans have high cholesterol, and an additional 63 million have borderline disease. Although the majority of the people with high cholesterol are adults, a growing number of young children and adolescents have high cholesterol as well. This is of special concern because hypercholesterolemia is a significant risk factor for heart disease.

Specifically, when there is too much cholesterol in your bloodstream, you can develop fatty deposits in your blood vessels, including your arteries, leading to a condition known as atherosclerosis. Atherosclerosis refers to the accumulation of fats, calcium, and other substances (plaque) in and on the artery walls that restricts blood flow and makes it difficult for the blood to carry the oxygen and nutrients from the heart to the rest of the body. If the plaques burst, they can cause a blood clot that can travel to the heart or brain. Restricted blood flow can lead to stroke, heart attack, or peripheral artery disease, which collectively are referred to as cardiovascular disease.

High cholesterol and atherosclerosis are both preventable and treatable, and efforts to do both should begin immediately, regardless of age. In fact, research shows evidence of atherosclerosis in teenagers and that plaque accumulation is found in 85 percent of adults older than 50.

Causes and Symptoms

High cholesterol is caused largely by lifestyle choices, including a high-fat, high-cholesterol diet, insufficient fiber in the diet, smoking, and lack of exercise, which can result in an accumulation of cholesterol plaque in the arteries and high blood pressure. Atherosclerosis is a silent disease, which means symptoms typically do not appear until the arteries narrow to a point that they choke off the blood flow and cause pain and a serious event, such as stroke. Other risk factors for atherosclerosis include stress, not eating enough fruits and vegetables, and excessive alcohol use.

How Supplements Can Help

- Garlic has been shown in some clinical trials to reduce cholesterol levels, prevent blood clots, and destroy plaque. Dosing: 900 mg daily standardized to 0.6 percent allicin. Children may take one-third to two-thirds of this dose, depending on their body weight.

- Green tea has been shown to significantly reduce total and LDL cholesterol. The adult dose of green tea extract is 300 to 400 mg daily. For children weighing 50 pounds, one-third of the adult dose is suggested; for those weighing 100 pounds, two-thirds of the dose is considered safe.

- Hawthorn contains the polyphenols rutin and quercetin, which are helpful in treating cardiovascular diseases. Hawthorn helps lower cholesterol levels and protect against the development of plaque. A suggested dose is 80 to 300 mg in capsules or tablets taken two to three times daily. For children weighing 50 pounds, one-third of the adult dose is suggested; those weighing 100 pounds can take two-thirds of the dose. Parents should consult their physician before giving children hawthorn for high cholesterol.

- Psyllium has been shown in many studies to help lower cholesterol. It pays to experiment with doses because psyllium is also used to treat both constipation and diarrhea. Begin with ½ teaspoon of psyllium seed in 8 ounces of warm water. You may gradually increase up to 2 teaspoons daily if you do not experience any discomfort. Mix well and drink quickly before it becomes too thick to swallow. If you use a commercial product that contains psyllium, follow the package instructions.

- Vitamin D: Most people are deficient in this sunshine vitamin. While having an adequate level of vitamin D is critical for many health reasons, one of those reasons is to prevent or slow the development of atherosclerosis, especially in people who have diabetes. It is helpful to have your vitamin D level checked so you know how much of the supplement you need to take to bring your levels up to between 50 and 80 ng/mL. For some people, this means taking 1,000 to 5,000 IU daily.

When to See a Doctor

If you are using nutritional supplements and/or herbal remedies to lower your cholesterol, it is a good idea to have your cholesterol levels checked periodically. Let your doctor know that you or your children are taking supplements to lower your cholesterol.

INFLAMMATORY BOWEL DISEASE

The term "inflammatory bowel disease" describes a group of intestinal disorders that impact the lives of more than 1 million people in the United States. The two most common types of inflammatory bowel disease are Crohn's disease and ulcerative colitis, and they can affect people of any age, although most cases first appear in people in mid-adolescence up to age 40.

Crohn's disease and ulcerative colitis share some characteristics, although they are not the same disease. Crohn's disease can affect the entire digestive tract, from the mouth to the anus, while ulcerative colitis is limited to the colon and rectum. The two conditions have some similar symptoms, but Crohn's disease is typically the more serious of the two. People who have inflammatory bowel disease usually experience a roller coaster of symptoms: When the inflammation is severe the disease causes symptoms, and when inflammation subsides the symptoms usually go away until something triggers the inflammation again.

Causes and Symptoms

The cause of inflammatory bowel disease is not known, but experts have some theories. Diet appears to play a part, as the vast majority of people who have the disease consume significant amounts of animal protein, processed foods, fat, and sugar. Some experts believe viruses, bacteria, parasites, or other microorganisms have a role. There is also evidence that the body's own tissues trigger an autoimmune response, which means the body attacks its own cells and damages the intestinal wall, causing bloody diarrhea and abdominal pain.

In Crohn's disease, inflammation and sores can occur anywhere along the digestive tract, although in most people they occur in the intestinal tract, which makes digestion difficult. Individuals who have Crohn's disease typically experience chronic diarrhea, weakness, pain, weight loss, and poor absorption of nutrients. People who have ulcerative colitis can experience painful diarrhea and bloody stools along with the other symptoms. Inflammatory bowel disease can also be accompanied by rashes and arthritis.

How Supplements Can Help

- NAC has been shown to relieve symptoms of inflammatory bowel disease, which is credited to its antioxidant powers. The suggested adult dose is 500 to 600 mg twice daily. Children may take one-quarter to one-half the adult dose.

- Probiotics: Numerous studies have shown that probiotics can relieve symptoms of both Crohn's disease and ulcerative colitis. Success has been observed with several different beneficial bacteria, including various Bifidobacterium and the probiotic yeast *Saccharomyces boulardii.*

- Slippery elm bark can help relieve intestinal inflammation. A suggested adult dose is two to three tablets or capsules each containing 400 to 500 mg three times daily. An alternative is slippery elm tea prepared by steeping 1 to 2 g of slippery elm bark in 8 ounces of boiled water for 10 minutes. For best results, drink 3 to 4 cups of tea daily. Children weighing 50 pounds can take one-third the adult oral supplement dose or drink 1 cup daily (several ounces each dose); those who weigh 100 pounds can take two-thirds the oral supplement dose or drink 2 cups daily. To sweeten the tea, you can use a little bit of cinnamon or ginger, both of which can also help the intestinal tract.

- Vitamin D: A recent study (January 2010) found that vitamin D supplements can help relieve symptoms of inflammatory bowel disease. Most people are deficient in this important vitamin, so taking more than the RDA may be necessary to help restore the body's level of this nutrient. For adults, 1,000 to 2,000 IU daily of a vitamin D supplement may be sufficient unless you undergo a vitamin D test that shows you are significantly deficient in this critical vitamin. In that case, your doctor may recommend a higher dose, 5,000 to 10,000 IU daily, for several months until the deficiency is resolved.

When to See a Doctor

Contact your physician if you see blood clots in your stool or if you experience any sudden episodes of fever, abdominal pain, and an urgent need to pass stool or gas.

INSOMNIA

When you can't fall asleep or you have trouble staying asleep, it can ruin your day. When it happens night after night, it can ruin your life, making it difficult to work, take care of your family, or do everyday activities, and it can also affect your health.

More than one-third of adults experience insomnia at some time, and up to 15 percent report having long-term insomnia. This sleep problem is more prevalent among older people and women. Although the rate of insomnia increases as a function of age, in most people insomnia is attributable to some medical condition.

But insomnia is not just for adults: Children and adolescents also experience difficulty sleeping. Lack of sufficient sleep can have a serious impact on young people's ability to do their schoolwork and participate in other activities.

How much sleep do people need? Generally, adults need seven to eight hours of sleep, while children between the ages of six and 12 need about 10 to 11 hours each night, and teens need about nine.

Causes and Symptoms

Insomnia is usually caused by a medical condition or use of a substance that affects the ability to sleep. Here are some common causes of insomnia.

- Stress: If you are worried about your job, school, health, or family, or if you have experienced stressful events such as a death or illness, divorce, or loss of a job, these may led to insomnia.

- Depression: When you are depressed, you may sleep too little or too much.

- Caffeine, nicotine, alcohol: Caffeine and nicotine are stimulants that can prevent you from falling asleep and staying asleep. Alcohol is a sedative that may help you fall asleep, but it prevents deeper stages of sleep and often makes you wake up in the middle of the night.

• Medications: Both over-the-counter and prescription drugs can interfere with sleep. Some of these include antidepressants, heart and blood pressure medications, allergy medications, and corticosteroids. Any medication that contains caffeine or other stimulants can disturb sleep.

• Medical conditions: Chronic respiratory conditions, chronic pain, the need to urinate often, and various other medical problems can cause or contribute to insomnia. If these medical concerns are addressed, your insomnia may be resolved.

• Eating: Going to bed with a full stomach can contribute to insomnia, as well as cause heartburn (see "Heartburn/GERD").

• Changes in schedule: If you are traveling or have changes to your work schedule, it can disrupt your circadian rhythms and make it difficult to sleep.

• Going to bed too late: This is a significant cause among children. Some parents have unrealistic expectations about how much sleep children need, or children are so over-scheduled or have so much homework or other activities that they stay awake much too late.

• Neurodevelopmental disorders: This is another cause of insomnia among children, including autism, mental retardation, and Asperger's syndrome.

Among older people, changes can occur that have a significant impact on sleep.

• Sleep pattern changes: Sleep tends to become less restful and refreshing as people age, because they spend more time in less restful stages of sleep. This can cause older people to sleep more lightly and thus they can wake up more often and easily.

• Less physical activity: When people become less active, they are more likely to take a daily nap, which can interfere with nighttime sleep, or just not feel as tired, even though they still need seven to eight hours of sleep.

• Changes in health: Older adults are more likely to experience painful conditions such as arthritis, restless legs, and back problems, as well as prostate conditions (men) and hot flashes (women).

• Increased medication use: Older adults tend to take more prescription drugs than younger people, which increases their chances of experiencing insomnia as a side effect.

Symptoms of insomnia include having trouble falling asleep, waking up and having trouble going back to sleep, waking up too early in the morning, feeling like you didn't get enough sleep, daytime drowsiness or anxiety, loss of the ability to concentrate during the day, and irritability.

How Supplements Can Help

• B vitamins can have a relaxing effect on the nerves. A combination of 50 to 100 mg daily of B_6, along with 25 mg of vitamin B_{12} and 100 mg of B_5, may be the answer to your insomnia if you are an adult.

• Chamomile is a classic herbal remedy for insomnia. Prepare a cup of chamomile tea in late afternoon and before bedtime. If you worry about having to get up during the night to urinate, you can try the tincture: 30 drops taken three times daily. Children who weigh 50 pounds can take one-third the dose and those who weigh 100 pounds can take two-thirds the dose.

• Magnesium deficiency or even low levels can cause insomnia, and low levels are common. A suggested dose for adults is 250 mg two to four times daily. The magnesium can be balanced with an equal amount of calcium.

• Melatonin is popular for promoting a sound night's sleep, especially if you travel across time zones or you work at night. A typical dose ranges from 1 mg up to 3 mg taken about 30 minutes before going to bed.

• Valerian can be effective once it "takes hold" in the body, which means you may have to take it for several weeks before you notice significant benefits. A suggested dose is 300 to 900 mg of valerian extract taken 30 minutes to two hours before bedtime.

When to See a Doctor

You should see a doctor about your insomnia if it lasts for longer than four weeks or if it disrupts your daily life and makes it difficult for you to function.

MIGRAINE

Between 25 and 30 million Americans experience the severe, often debilitating head pain known as migraine at some point in their lives. This condition does not only affect adults: About 50 percent of people get their first migraine before they reach the age of 20, and it is estimated that up to 10 percent of children between the ages of five and 15 experience migraine. Before puberty, girls and boys get migraine in about equal numbers, but once puberty sets in, migraines affect girls three times more often than boys, and this 3-to-1 ratio continues throughout adulthood.

Migraines can appear in two main forms: classic and common. They are similar except for the presence of an aura stage in the classic form, which affects about 20 to 30 percent of people who get migraine.

Causes and Symptoms

Migraine is classified as a vascular headache, which means it is caused by changes to the blood vessels. In migraine, these changes occur at the base of the brain, causing the vessels to restrict blood flow and then expand, sending a burst of blood to the brain and resulting in intense pain.

The question is, what triggers the changes in the blood vessels? People who suffer with migraine report many different factors that can set off an attack, including eating certain foods, stress, hormonal changes (migraines are more common before and during a menstrual period), exposure to chemicals or air pollutants, smoking, and getting too little or too much sleep. Migraine has also been associated with a magnesium deficiency, changes in barometric pressure, and eyestrain.

If your migraine pain is preceded by visual disturbances such as spots or wavy lines, or you experience pins and needles anywhere in your body, these are symptoms of an aura, which typically appear about 30 to 60 minutes before the pain. The head pain in both forms of migraine usually begins as throbbing on one side of the head and moves to the forehead, temples, jaw, top of the head, or one nostril. Other symptoms include hypersensitivity to light or sounds, constipation or diarrhea, nausea and/or vomiting, muscle aches, chills, muscle spasms in the back and neck, and oversensitivity to touch.

How Supplements Can Help

- Butterbur has proved to be effective in several studies, reducing the frequency of migraine by nearly 50 percent compared with placebo at 26 percent. A suggested dose is 75 mg twice a day. Children who weigh 50 pounds can take one-third the dose while those weighing 100 pounds can take two-thirds the dose.

- The B vitamin niacin taken during an aura episode can stop a migraine attack in some individuals. That's because the vitamin causes the blood vessels to constrict rapidly. A suggested dose is 100 mg as soon as symptoms of an aura occur. Children may take one-quarter to one-half the dose.

- Feverfew is an herb that can be effective both to prevent and treat migraine. For prevention, the suggested dose is 125 mg of dried herb daily, standardized at 0.25 to 0.5 percent panthenolide (an active ingredient). To help ward off an acute attack, take 475 mg as soon as you detect symptoms. Repeat the same dose every four hours, but do not take more than 1,500 mg within a 24-hour period. Although there are no definitive studies of feverfew in children, you may consider giving a child who weighs 50 pounds one-third the adult dose, and a 100-pound child two-thirds the adult dose.

- Magnesium supplements can help prevent migraine in people who have low magnesium levels, which is not uncommon among migraineurs. Magnesium can reduce the expansion and constriction of blood vessels. A suggested dose is 400 to 600 mg daily for adults, and one-quarter to one-half the dose for children.

When to See a Doctor

You should call your doctor immediately if you experience any of the following: unusually severe head pain, a migraine that does not respond to treatment and lasts longer than three days, migraine accompanied by a fever of 102°F or higher, slurred speech, blurry vision, weakness, or head pain that increases when you bend your chin to your chest.

PEPTIC ULCERS

Open sores that develop in the lining of the stomach, esophagus, or duodenum are called peptic ulcers. The American College of Gastroenterology says that about 20 million Americans can expect to have an ulcer during their lives. For most people that experience happens when they are adults, but children can develop peptic ulcers too.

Causes and Symptoms

Clinicians used to think that spicy and/or fatty foods caused peptic ulcers, but in most cases, the cause of ulcers is *Helicobacter pylori,* a type of bacteria that weakens the protective coating of the stomach and the first part of the intestine and allows damaging digestive juices to erode the lining. About 20 percent of people older than 40 have *H. pylori* lurking in their digestive tract, and this is where the spicy foods come in. Some people who have *H. pylori* will go on to develop peptic ulcers, and the triggers may include spicy or fatty foods, coffee, stress, alcohol, or smoking.

The second most important cause of peptic ulcers is longterm use of nonsteroidal anti-inflammatory drugs (NSAIDs). These substances block prostaglandins, which are responsible for maintaining blood flow and protecting the stomach. Some people can use NSAIDs without a problem, yet others develop problems, including peptic ulcers.

Symptoms of peptic ulcer in both children and adults

include burning pain in the abdomen between the breastbone and belly button, nausea, vomiting, weight loss, blood in vomit or stool, pain two to three hours after eating, and poor appetite.

How Supplements Can Help

Because the main cause of peptic ulcers is *H. pylori* infection, getting rid of the bacteria is one goal of treatment while relieving symptoms is the other. Although symptoms are reduced as the antibiotics take effect, nutritional and herbal supplements can help as well. You should also consider making some lifestyle changes if you have habits that are contributing to your ulcers.

- Aloe vera juice (not gel) can provide symptom relief. Drink ⅓ cup three times daily. Children can be given one-third to two-thirds the dose, depending on their weight. Truthfully, most children are not fond of aloe vera juice, and unless you attempt to disguise it in juice or another beverage, they probably will not drink it. Fortunately, there are other remedies you can try.

- Cranberry may inhibit the growth of *H. pylori* in the stomach. Try taking 400 mg tablets twice daily. Children can be given one-third to two-thirds the dose, depending on their weight.

- Licorice (DGL: deglycyrrhizinated) may help protect the stomach against damage from NSAIDs. An adult dose is 250 to 500 mg three times daily of standardized extract taken one hour before or two hours after a meal. Children who weigh 50 pounds can take one-third the dose, and those weighing 100 pounds can take two-thirds the dose.

- Peppermint may relieve symptoms of peptic ulcer. A suggested dose is one standardized, enteric-coated tablet two to three times daily. Each tablet should contain 0.2 mL peppermint oil. Enteric-coated forms are important, because they help avoid heartburn.

- Probiotic supplement that contains *Lactobacillus acidophilus* and other species. Take 5 to 10 billion CFUs daily. Children can take one-quarter to one-half the dose. Probiotics are especially important if you or your child are taking antibiotics against *H. pylori* because the drug can destroy the beneficial bacteria in the intestinal tract while probiotics can help restore them.

When to See a Doctor

If you experience any of the following symptoms, call your doctor immediately: vomiting blood or substances that look like coffee grounds, blood in your stool or black, tarry stools, or a sudden increase in abdominal pain or sharpness in the degree of pain.

PREMENSTRUAL SYNDROME

Premenstrual syndrome (PMS) is a disorder characterized by hormonal changes that trigger uncomfortable and/or disruptive symptoms in many women for up to two weeks before menstruation. It is estimated that 40 million women suffer with PMS, and that more than 5 million need medical treatment for the significant changes in behavior and mood that they experience.

Causes and Symptoms

The exact cause of PMS and all of its symptoms are unknown. Experts are not sure why some women experience very mild symptoms while others suffer a great deal. The general consensus is that PMS and its symptoms stem from neurochemical changes within the brain. The influence of hormones has only recently been appreciated in PMS.

What happens is, estrogen levels begin to rise after menstruation and peak around mid-cycle, which is when ovulation occurs. Estrogen levels then drop rapidly, slowly rise, and then fall again before menstruation. Symptoms often taper off during menstruation and stay away until the whole cycle begins again about two weeks before the next menstrual period.

More than 150 symptoms have been attributed to PMS, entirely too many to list here. The most common complaints include feeling "out of control," anxiety, depressing crying jags, headache, fluid retention, and fatigue. Symptoms can vary in intensity from month to month, and may not even occur in some months. Some of the other symptoms may include backache, nausea and vomiting, tender breasts, muscle spasms, constipation, irritability, panic attacks, and reduced libido.

How Supplements Can Help

- B vitamins as a group help the nervous system and can also relieve breast tenderness. Take one high-potency B complex supplement daily. You can also include an additional 100 mg vitamin B_6 for extra relief from fluid retention.

- Chasteberry is one of the most effective herbal remedies for PMS because it is a potent anti-inflammatory. Studies show this herb can reduce breast tenderness, irritability, depression, and headache. The suggested dose is 200 mg of the berry standardized to 0.5 percent agnuside. You can also take the tincture or extract mixed with water, 10 to 30 drops per drink taken three times daily. Chasteberry tea can be made from the ripe berries (a teaspoon) in 8 ounces of boiling water, steeped for 10 to 15 minutes and enjoyed three times daily.

- Dandelion root or leaf tea can relieve bloating, water retention, tender breasts, and muscle spasms. Two cups of dandelion tea daily are suggested. Use 1 to 2 teaspoons of dried dandelion leaves or one teaspoon of dried root per cup of tea. Allow the dried dandelion to steep in hot water for 5 to 10 minutes. If you prefer, you can take two capsules (400–500 mg each) of dried dandelion three times daily with food.

- Magnesium can reduce bloating, breast tenderness, weight gain, and mood changes. A suggested dose is 360 mg three times daily starting from day 15 to the start of the menstrual period.

- Valerian has dual powers: It can relieve menstrual cramping and relieve emotional stress and irritability. As a tea, steep 1½ to 3 g of the root for 5 to 10 minutes in 6 ounces of boiling water. For cramping, take ½ teaspoon of the tincture every two to three hours until symptoms resolve.

When to See a Doctor

If you have tried several different supplements and have changed lifestyle habits that can contribute to PMS symptoms, and you are still feeling terrible; if your PMS symptoms regularly disrupt your life; if you feel out of control because of your PMS symptoms; and/or if significant symptoms (e.g., depression, mood swings, anxiety, crying) do not stop after a couple of days of your menstrual period, it's time to see your doctor.

SHINGLES

Shingles (herpes zoster) is a viral infection that attacks the nerve roots. It is most common in older adults and people who have a weak immune system because of illness, use of certain medications, stress, or injury. An estimated 1 million people per year suffer with shingles, and most of them get the condition only once. Children do not get shingles.

Anyone who has had chicken pox can get shingles. Your chances of getting shingles increase significantly if you are older than 50, if you have an autoimmune disease (e.g., rheumatoid arthritis, fibromyalgia, type 1 diabetes), or if you have any other health problem that weakens the immune system. If you have never had chicken pox and have never gotten a vaccine for the disease, you should avoid touching anyone who has shingles or chicken pox. Individuals who are at least 60 years old can get a vaccine that may prevent shingles or make it less painful if they do get it.

Causes and Symptoms

Shingles occurs when the virus that causes chicken pox "wakes up" after it has been dormant for years. That's because after a person has chicken pox, the virus hibernates in the nerve roots. This virus stays dormant forever in some people, but it reemerges when disease, stress, or aging weakens the immune system. Although you cannot catch shingles from someone who has the condition, a person with a shingles rash can spread chicken pox to another person who has not had this disease and who has not received the chicken pox vaccine.

Symptoms of shingles occur in stages. At first, people often experience a headache or are sensitive to light. Some people feel like they have the flu but they do not have a fever. Over time, itching, tingling, or pain develops in certain areas of the body, especially the trunk. A rash may occur a few days later, and it usually develops into clusters of blisters that fill with fluid and then crust over. The blisters usually heal in about two to four weeks, and they may leave scars. Other symptoms may include dizziness, long-term pain, facial rash, changes in vision, or weakness.

In about 20 percent of people who get shingles, the pain lingers on and on for months or even years after the rash and blisters have disappeared. This condition is known as postherpetic neuralgia. Symptoms include stabbing pain where the shingles had occurred, extreme sensitivity to touch and temperature change, and headache.

How Supplements Can Help

- The amino acid lysine prevents the absorption of arginine, which the shingles virus needs to stay active. A suggested dose of lysine is 1,000 mg three times daily until symptoms disappear.

- Capsaicin is a common natural remedy for postherpetic neuralgia and shingles. Capsaicin cream can be applied to the affected areas two to four times daily. A typical dosage is 0.025 percent capsaicin cream. It may take several weeks before you notice a significant benefit from this treatment. For shingles, you can also mix a small amount of cayenne pepper and aloe vera gel and apply to the affected areas.

- Echinacea provides anti-viral and immune-boosting benefits for people who have shingles. The suggested dose is ½ teaspoon extract taken three times daily, or 300-mg capsules taken 10 times daily.

- Goldenseal has both antimicrobial and immune-boosting properties. You can take 500 mg to 2,000 mg three times daily of the dried root or ½ to 1 teaspoon of liquid extract three times daily.

- MSM can help with pain relief. A dose of 1,000 mg at least twice daily is suggested.

When to See a Doctor

You may want to contact your doctor if you experience dizziness and/or weakness along with shingles, the rash is on your face, you notice changes in your vision, or if the rash spreads extensively.

STREP/SORE THROAT

It would be hard to find someone who has never had a sore throat. This symptom or condition is so common, it is one of the main reasons people go to a doctor. Yet in most cases a sore throat is caused by a virus that will go away by itself, and a visit to the doctor is not necessary. When bacteria are involved, medical treatment may be needed. In either case, however, nutrients and herbs can provide relief.

Causes and Symptoms

The most common viruses that can cause a sore throat are the common cold and flu, while strep is the most common bacterial cause of a sore throat. A sore throat can also be caused by allergies, dry air, GERD, air pollutants, muscle strain (shouting, overuse of the voice), and smoking.

Symptoms of a sore throat are dry scratchiness and painful swallowing. If your sore throat is caused by a strep infection, then symptoms can include white patches or pus on your throat or tonsils, an inability to swallow, severe throat pain, headache, vomiting, swollen tonsils, and a high fever.

How Supplements Can Help

- Chamomile tea is a favorite herbal remedy for sore throats. Steep one teaspoon of dried chamomile in 8 ounces of hot water for 5 to 10 minutes and drink 2 to 3 cups daily. Children can enjoy one-third to two-thirds of this dose, depending on their body weight.

- Cinnamon can be helpful for a sore throat associated with a cold or flu. Add one teaspoon of powdered cinnamon to a cup of boiled water and stir in 1 teaspoon of honey. Take this remedy two to three times a day. Children can take one-third to two-thirds of this herbal remedy, depending on body weight.

- Echinacea and goldenseal combination can help eliminate the infection and boost the immune system. Add 10 to 15 drops of tincture of each herb to a small amount of water and take four times daily for two days, then one dose three times daily for two to three days. Children can take one-third to two-thirds of this dose depending on body weight.

- Licorice can soothe the throat, and kids like this remedy. Add 1 tablespoon of licorice root to 8 ounces of boiling water and simmer for 10 minutes. Let it cool before drinking. Adults can take 1 to 2 cups daily; children can drink one-third to two-thirds of this dose, depending on their weight.

- Slippery elm tea or lozenges can help a sore throat. To prepare the tea, pour 16 ounces of boiling water over 2 tablespoons of powdered bark and allow it to steep for 3 to 5 minutes. Drink 3 cups daily for adults; children may take one-third to two-thirds of this dose, depending on body weight. If you choose lozenges, follow the package instructions.

When to See a Doctor

You or your child should see a doctor if any of the following occur:

- The sore throat is severe and lasts longer than seven days
- Swallowing or breathing is difficult
- An infant has a fever greater than 101°F, or an older child or adult has a fever greater than 103°F
- The lymph nodes are tender or swollen in the neck

- Pus or white patches have developed in the throat
- Hoarseness or a cough develops and lasts more than two weeks
- There is blood in saliva or phlegm
- Excessive drooling (in young children)

URINARY TRACT INFECTIONS

Every year, 8 to 10 million Americans suffer from a urinary tract infection, a bacterial infection that attacks the bladder, ureters (the tube that transports urine from the kidney to the bladder), and the urethra (the tube that carries urine out of the body). Urinary tract infections are the second most common infection after respiratory infection. They are most common among women, although they also affect men and, to a lesser degree, children.

There are three types of urinary tract infection, and each has its own symptoms. When the infection is limited to the urethra, the condition is called urethritis, and when it reaches the bladder it is known as cystitis. If this infection is not treated promptly, it can spread to the kidneys, resulting in a more serious condition called pyelonephritis.

Causes and Symptoms

A urinary tract infection develops when bacteria enter the urinary tract through the urethra and begin to reproduce in the bladder. In urethritis, bacteria travel from the anus to the urethra. In many cases the bacteria are *Escherichia coli,* which are commonly found in the gastrointestinal tract. However, because the female urethra is very close to the vagina, sexually transmitted disease such as gonorrhea and chlamydia are also possible causes of urethritis.

Cystitis is also usually caused by *E. coli.* All women are susceptible to cystitis because the urethra is very close to the anus and thus provides a short distance for the bacteria to travel.

Generally, urinary tract infections are characterized by a

frequent urge to urinate, passing only small amounts of urine, painful urination, and cloudy or milking-looking urine. Burning with urination is a symptom of urethritis, while pelvic pressure, discomfort in the lower abdomen, and low-grade fever are common with cystitis. If the disease has progressed to pyelonephritis, symptoms usually include high fever, chills, pain in the upper back and side, nausea, and vomiting.

How Supplements Can Help

- Cranberries have been used for more than 100 years to prevent and treat urinary tract infections. Research suggests that substances in cranberries called proanthocyanins prevent bacteria from sticking to the walls of the urinary tract. Studies also indicate that cranberry tablets are more effective than the juice. A recommended dose is 300 to 400 mg capsules, six times daily. If you prefer the juice, drink at least 3 ounces of pure, unsweetened cranberry juice daily. For children, use one-third to two-thirds of the adult dose, depending on body weight.

- Garlic tea (or garlic broth if that sounds more appealing) contains potent bacteria-killing compounds. Peel two to three cloves of fresh garlic, mash them well, and let them steep in hot water for five minutes. In a pinch, you can use one teaspoon of garlic powder stirred well into hot water.

- Goldenseal is a natural enemy of the *E. coli* bacteria that cause many cases of urinary tract infections. The suggested dose is 500 to 1,000 mg of goldenseal root extract once daily for up to seven days. Children who weigh 50 pounds may take one-third the dose, while those weighing 100 pounds can take two-thirds.

- Vitamin C can make your bladder more resistant to clinging bacteria and is recommended by some clinicians to fight urinary tract infections. The suggested dose for adults is 1,000 to 1,400 mg daily. Children may be given one-quarter to one-half the adult dose.

When to See a Doctor

If you or your child experience constant pressure or pain in the abdomen, side, or lower back, or you have fever, nausea, vomiting, or chills, contact your doctor. The infection may have spread to your kidneys, and this requires immediate attention.

VAGINITIS

Vaginitis is a general term for several different types of vaginal infections, each of which is caused by a different organism. All types of vaginitis involve inflammation of the vagina that can result in vaginal discharge, pain, and itching. The three most common types of vaginitis are caused by yeast, bacteria, and protozoa, and of the three, yeast vaginitis can be treated without a physician, so we focus on this variety. Vaginal yeast infections also affect about 70 percent of women at least once during their lifetime, and many women have two or more episodes.

If you believe you have vaginitis, it is necessary to learn which type you have so it can be treated properly. The test can be done quickly in a clinic or doctor's office. One clue that a vaginal infection is not caused by yeast is that the vaginal discharge may be gray or yellow-green and have an odor. However, it is still best to get an accurate diagnosis because, left untreated or mistreated, all types of vaginitis can spread up the genital tract and cause pelvic inflammatory disease, an infection of the fallopian tubes, or other complications.

Causes and Symptoms

Yeast vaginitis is most often caused by a microscopic fungus called *Candida albicans*. Yeast infections occur when an internal or external factor changes the normal environment of the vagina, triggering excessive growth of the fungus. Risk factors for yeast vaginitis include hormonal changes associated with pregnancy or use of birth control pills, use of medications such as antibiotics or steroids, and uncontrolled diabetes. Use of feminine hygiene products, bubble baths, and tight-fitting clothing can increase your susceptibility to infection.

Symptoms of yeast vaginitis include vaginal itching or irritation, pain during intercourse, painful urination, light vaginal bleeding, and a change in the color, odor, or amount of vaginal discharge. The discharge may look like cottage cheese.

How Supplements Can Help

- An echinacea, goldenseal, and tea tree oil douche may relieve symptoms and eliminate the infections. Combine 10 drops of echinacea extract, 10 drops of goldenseal extract, and six drops of tea tree oil mixed in 2 cups of water. Douche with this herbal remedy once or twice daily for five days, then once a day for five more days.

- Cinnamon tea is a potent antifungal remedy. To prepare the tea, add 8 to 10 broken cinnamon sticks to 4 cups of boiling water. Simmer for 5 minutes, then steep for an additional 45 minutes. Drink 1 to 2 cups daily until the infection has completely disappeared.

- Garlic is a powerful antifungal agent. Take 500 mg garlic extract three times daily for seven to ten days.

- Probiotics can help restore a healthy balance of microorganisms in the vagina and intestinal tract.

Suggested dose is 16 billion CFUs of a multi-species probiotic supplement with each meal for five days, followed by 11 billion CFUs with each meal for an additional five days, then 5.5 billion CFUs per meal until the symptoms are gone.

• Vitamin E can be applied topically or inserted into the vagina for symptom relief. Vitamin E oil can be used to soothe the vagina and vulva; apply once or twice daily for three to 14 days. You can also insert a vitamin E suppository daily until symptoms resolve.

When to See a Doctor

If your infection does not improve after several days of treating it yourself, or if you get recurring vaginal yeast infections every few months, contact your doctor. You should also see a doctor if you have vaginitis and you are pregnant or if you are experiencing abdominal or pelvic pain.

PART III

Natural Supplements for You and Your Family

Part 3 consists of two sections: 16 entries for nutritional supplements, followed by 28 entries for herbal supplements. Each entry contains information about how to use the supplement for specific ailments, the majority of which we discussed in detail in Part 2, so feel free to refer back whenever you need to. Suggested dosages are provided for children (when applicable) and adults, and you are encouraged to check with your healthcare provider or other knowledgeable professional about taking any supplements, especially when they are taken by children, individuals who have a chronic illness, or women who are pregnant or breastfeeding.

NUTRITIONAL SUPPLEMENTS

AMINO ACIDS

Amino acids are substances that are used to build protein molecules. The body makes proteins from 20 amino acids, eight of which are called "essential" because the body cannot manufacture them. This means they must be obtained from the diet or supplements. The remaining 12 amino acids are produced in the body. For optimal health, it is best to maintain a balance among all the amino acids, although sometimes it is desirable to take an additional amount of one or more amino acids to treat specific symptoms or conditions.

Two of the amino acids produced by the body (arginine, glutamine) and two that are essential (lysine, methionine) are sometimes used to treat conditions that we cover in this book. Arginine is popular among bodybuilders because it has muscle-building properties. Foods that are rich in arginine include chocolate, peanuts, nuts, various seeds, and peas. Glutamine is the most abundant amino acid found in muscles. Food sources include beef, chicken, beans, and fish.

Lysine is important for proper growth and appears to help the body absorb calcium. This amino acid can be found in beans, dairy products, potatoes, and brewer's yeast. Methionine is a potent antioxidant and a good source of sulfur. It is found mainly in eggs, nuts, seeds, and some fish.

What Are the Benefits?

Lysine is very effective in treating sores caused by the herpes simplex virus, and by extension it is also useful in treating shingles, which is caused by a herpes virus. Many healthcare providers recommend using lysine along with antiviral medication for shingles. Lysine is also used to treat canker sores.

Arginine changes into nitric oxide, which causes blood vessels to relax. This makes arginine a treatment option for men who have erectile dysfunction, as well as individuals who have coronary artery disease or heart failure. People who have infections or burns may need to take arginine bcause it promotes healing.

Both methionine and glutamine are found in great levels in muscle and are used together to treat symptoms of gout. Methionine helps detoxify harmful substances from the body, while glutamine helps maintain the proper acid/alkaline balance in the body and promotes a healthy digestive tract.

How Much Should I Take?

Amino acids are available both individually and in mixed (combined) forms as powders, capsules, and liquids. A typical dose of lysine is 500 to 1,000 mg three times daily. A common dose of arginine is 2 to 3 g three times daily. A typical daily dose of methionine is 12 mg per kilogram of body weight (which equals about 840 mg for a 150-pound person). No standard dose has been established for glutamine. For treatment of gout, a common dose is 500 mg four times daily.

Cautionary Tales

Arginine can promote the growth of the herpes virus, so it should not be taken by people who have genital sores or cold sores. Lysine should not be taken with milk or dairy products. Use of lysine may raise cholesterol levels, and it can cause abdominal pain if taken at very high doses (more than 10 grams daily). Glutamine should not be taken if you suffer from seizures, are allergic to MSG, or if you have severe liver disease. Methionine does not appear to cause side effects when taken at suggested doses. Do not take amino acids if you are pregnant or breastfeeding.

B VITAMINS/B-COMPLEX

The B vitamins are a family of eight water-soluble nutrients that play a critical role in cell metabolism. At one time the B vitamins were believed to be just one vitamin, but research eventually revealed that they are chemically distinct substances that often appear in the same foods. The B vitamins are thus often taken together as a B-complex supplement because although each of the members has its own unique properties, they also work together in various combinations to support and enhance healing and health.

The main members of the B vitamin family are thiamin (B_1), riboflavin (B_2), niacin or niacinamide (B_3), pantothenic acid (B_5), pyridoxine (B_6), biotin (B_7), folic acid (B_9), and cobalamins (B_{12}). All eight members of the B vitamin family are found in a B-complex supplement, along with several other nutrients that are like "cousins" to the main B vitamins. The box on page 68 shows a typical B-complex supplement, although the B-complex supplement you choose may have somewhat different dosages and/or fewer, the same, or more of the "cousins."

What Are the Benefits?

Overall, the B vitamins support and increase the metabolism rate, maintain healthy muscle tone and skin, enhance nervous system and immune system functions, and promote the growth and division of cells. Each individual B vitamin may have specific features that make it important in the treatment of a certain symptom or disease.

For example, both folic acid and vitamin B_{12} are used to treat anemia that is caused by a deficiency of either of these vitamins, while niacin is effective in the treatment of migraine. In many cases, however, a B-complex supplement can be helpful in treating symptoms and conditions as varied as acne, ADHD, breast cancer, gout, insomnia, and premenstrual syndrome.

How Much Should I Take?

The recommended daily allowance (RDA) for each of the B vitamins is provided in the table in Chapter 3. Suggested doses for specific symptoms or medical conditions are provided in the appropriate entries in Part 2.

Cautionary Tales

The B vitamins are water soluble, so they do not build up in the body and reach toxic levels that could cause health problems. In fact, the therapeutic range (the amounts considered to be safe to take for specific ailments) for each of the B vitamins is many times their RDA. For example, the RDA for thiamin is 1.5 mg, and the therapeutic range is 50 to 1,000 mg. Therefore, you would have to take more than 70 times the RDA before you consumed a "dangerous" level of thiamin. Although the symptoms of overdose differ for each B vitamin, some common ones many of them share are nausea, vomiting, headache, severe fatigue, dizziness, and heart palpitations. If you have any reason to believe you or someone else has taken massive amounts of B vitamins, contact your doctor or seek medical help immediately.

COENZYME Q_{10}

Coenzyme Q_{10} (CoQ10) is a compound found in the energy-producing portion of the cell called the mitochondria. CoQ10 is a key player in the making of adenosine triphosphate (ATP), which is the cell's main energy source and the substance that drives numerous biological processes, such as muscle contraction and protein production.

Coenzyme Q_{10} is found in oily fish, organ meats, and whole grains, or can be taken as a supplement.

What Are the Benefits?

CoQ10 is a potent antioxidant, which means it seeks out and destroys free radicals. Free radicals are molecules that damage cells in the body and thus can cause cancer and other diseases as well as contribute to aging. Antioxidants can help prevent and treat these conditions. CoQ10 has proved beneficial in the treatment of a variety of symptoms and conditions, including high blood pressure, inflammatory bowel disease, periodontal disease, fatigue, and diabetes.

How Much Should I Take?

CoQ10 is available as soft gel capsules, hard shell capsules, and tablets. A typical dose for adults is 30 to 200 mg daily. The body can absorb the soft gels better than the other capsules or tablets, and the supplement is better utilized by the body if it is taken at night. CoQ10 is fat-soluble so you should take it with a meal that contains fat. Talk to your doctor before giving a CoQ10 supplement to children younger than 18.

Cautionary Tales

Coenzyme Q10 is generally safe and causes no significant side effects, except occasional stomach distress. Because its safety during pregnancy and breastfeeding is unknown, it should not be taken during these times. If you are taking any of the following medications, talk to your doctor before taking CoQ10: blood thinners (e.g., warfarin, clopidigrel), timolol, blood pressure medications (e.g., diltiazem, metoprolol, enalapril), daunorubicin, doxorubicin, cholesterol-lowering drugs (e.g., atorvastatin, lovastatin), and tricyclic antidepressants (e.g., amitriptyline, imipramine).

GLUCOSAMINE AND CHONDROITIN

Glucosamine and chondroitin are substances produced naturally in the body, where they have a strong association with cartilage, the connective tissue that cushions the joints. Glucosamine plays a major role in building cartilage, while chondroitin helps to keep cartilage healthy by absorbing fluid into the connective tissue.

What Are the Benefits?

Glucosamine and chondroitin are often, but not always, used together to treat arthritis, specifically osteoarthritis. Both supplements have been shown to reduce the pain associated with osteoarthritis and may also promote the repair or growth of new cartilage. Studies also indicate that these supplements may help reduce joint swelling and stiffness and improve function in people who have hip or knee osteoarthritis.

How Much Should I Take?

Most studies indicate that patients need to take glucosamine and chondroitin for about two months before the supplements are effective, although some improvement may be evident sooner. Because there are no significant food sources of glucosamine or chondroitin, supplements are the only way to get these substances.

Most glucosamine supplements are made from chitin, the hard outer shells of crabs and other crustaceans, although some manufacturers make other forms for people who are allergic to shellfish. Glucosamine is available as glucosamine sulfate, glucosamine hydrochloride, and n-acetyl glucosamine, and these are available as tablets, capsules, or a powder.

Many chondroitin supplements are made from cow cartilage, although some are made from algae. Chondroitin is sold as chondroitin sulfate in capsules or tablets. Glucosamine and chondroitin are often found together in a single supplement.

The suggested daily dose of glucosamine is 500 mg three times daily for 30 to 90 days. You can also take it as a single 1,500 mg dose. The dose for chondroitin is 400 mg three times daily or 600 mg twice daily.

Cautionary Tales

Manganese is sometimes an added ingredient in glucosamine/chondroitin supplements. Because the total amount of manganese you consume daily should not exceed 11 mg and some glucosamine/chondroitin products may contain more, it is best to purchase these supplements without manganese.

Glucosamine and chondroitin are both considered to be safe. Side effects are generally mild and may include stomach upset, heartburn, indigestion, bloating, and diarrhea. If side effects occur, take the supplement with food. Glucosamine sulfate may contain high levels of potassium or sodium, so check the label before taking glucosamine if you are on a salt-restricted diet or you take potassium-sparing diuretics.

If you are using nonsteroidal anti-inflammatory drugs (NSAIDs), taking glucosamine may reduce the dose of NSAIDs that you need. Glucosamine may also alter the dose for blood sugar lowering medications and insulin if you have diabetes.

IRON

Iron is a critical part of many proteins and enzymes that maintain good health. This mineral is necessary for a number of critical functions, including carrying oxygen to the tissues throughout the body. In fact, nearly two-thirds of the iron in the body is located in hemoglobin, the protein in red blood cells that carries the oxygen. Iron is also essential for cell growth and development.

Dietary iron is available in two forms: heme and nonheme. Heme iron is derived from hemoglobin and is found in animal foods, such as red meat, fish, and poultry. Iron in plants such as lentils and beans is called nonheme iron. This is also the form of iron that is added to iron-enriched foods.

What Are the Benefits?

An adequate intake of iron helps prevent anemia, a condition characterized by fatigue, weakness, slow mental functioning, hypersensitivity to changes in temperature, and reduced immune function, making you more likely to develop an ailment or disease. Iron supplementation can help people who have a greater need for iron, those who tend to lose more iron, and people who do not absorb iron normally. These individuals include pregnant women, preterm and low birth weight infants, adolescent girls, women who have heavy menstrual losses, and people with gastrointestinal disorders who do not absorb iron normally.

How Much Should I Take?

The RDA for iron can be seen in the chart in Chapter 3 (p. 58–59). Basically, males need 7 to 11 mg and females need 7 to 18 mg. Females begin to require a higher amount of iron during adolescence, when menstruation typically begins, and that greater need continues until menopause. Because taking too much iron can cause problems (see "Cautionary Tales"), you should talk to your doctor before you or your family takes iron supplements.

Iron supplements are available in two forms: ferrous and ferric. Ferrous iron salts (ferrous fumarate, ferrous sulfate, ferrous gluconate) are best absorbed by the body. Elemental iron is the amount of iron in a supplement that is available for absorption and is less likely to cause constipation, a common side effect of iron supplementation.

Cautionary Tales

Too much iron can result in symptoms of overdose (e.g., nausea, vomiting, diarrhea, constipation) and even death. The tolerable upper limit of iron is only 40 mg for children and 45 mg for adults. Therefore it is important to pay attention to the amount of iron that may be in any supplements you and your family take.

MAGNESIUM

Magnesium is the fourth most abundant mineral in the body. About half of the body's magnesium is found in bone, while the other half is inside cells of body tissues and organs. Although only 1 percent of magnesium is found in blood, that 1 percent is critical to maintain for health.

Food sources of magnesium include green vegetables such as spinach, as well as legumes, nuts, seeds, and whole, unrefined grains. Processed white flour and products made from it are poor sources, because the magnesium-rich germ and bran have been removed.

What Are the Benefits?

Magnesium is a mineral that is needed for more than 300 biochemical reactions in the body. Among its many tasks, magnesium helps maintain normal muscle and nerve function, keeps heart rhythm steady, supports bone strength, and maintains a healthy immune system. Magnesium is helpful in preventing and managing conditions such as ADHD, anemia, asthma, bronchitis, constipation, diabetes, gout, migraine, and PMS.

How Much Should I Take?

The RDA for magnesium for each age group can be seen in the chart in Chapter 3 (pp. 58–59). Generally, males 14 years and older need 400 to 420 mg daily and females need 310 to 360 mg, with slightly higher levels during pregnancy and breastfeeding. Magnesium deficiency is not uncommon, but many people do not show signs of low magnesium. Early symptoms can include loss of appetite, nausea, vomiting, fatigue, and weakness.

Older adults are at increased risk for magnesium deficiency for several reasons. One, they are less able to absorb magnesium while at the same time they excrete more in their urine. Two, they are less likely than younger adults to consume enough magnesium in their diet. And three, older adults are more likely to be taking drugs that interact with magnesium (see "Cautionary Tales"). Therefore, it is important to make sure older adults get an adequate amount of this important mineral.

Cautionary Tales

Use of loop and thiazide diuretics, which are used to treat high blood pressure and heart disease, can increase the body's excretion of magnesium and lead to a magnesium deficiency. Long-term use of antineoplastic drugs can also increase magnesium excretion.

MELATONIN

Melatonin is a hormone that is produced and secreted by the pineal gland in the brain. Many people associate melatonin with insomnia and sleep, and that's right on target because one of this hormone's major jobs is to maintain the body's circadian rhythm, the 24-hour internal clock that helps regulate your wake/sleep cycle. It also has a role in the timing and release of female reproductive hormones, so it is associated with menstruation and menopause.

Melatonin's activity is dependant on light. When it is dark, the body produces more melatonin; when it is light, production declines. Therefore, if you or your children are exposed to bright lights at night, it will disrupt the body's normal melatonin cycles—and your sleep as well! (Hint: Young children have the highest levels of nighttime melatonin. Get your child used to sleeping in the dark, with a small night light only. Sleeping with the lights on will disturb their sleep habits.)

What Are the Benefits?

Melatonin's biggest claim to fame is its ability to help people sleep better and to combat insomnia. Specifically, it can reduce the amount of time it takes to fall asleep, increase the number of hours you do sleep, and improve daytime alertness. It is also effective in helping people who experience jet lag or who work night shifts. Melatonin also appears to promote sleep in some children who have attention deficit hyperactivity disorder (ADHD), but it has no impact on other ADHD symptoms.

Melatonin also may have a role in cancer. Levels of melatonin tend to be lower in women who have breast cancer than those without the disease. Laboratory research suggests that melatonin may slow breast cancer cell growth, and that it may also improve the effects of some chemotherapy drugs used in the treatment of breast cancer. In one study, women who were taking tamoxifen and not experiencing any improvement began taking melatonin. More than 28 percent of the women had a modest reduction in tumor size after taking the hormone. There is also some evidence that melatonin may help strengthen the immune system.

How Much Should I Take?

We recommend that you begin with a very low dose, one that is close to the amount the body makes naturally, which is less than 0.3 mg per day. Low doses appear to be just as effective as higher doses, so why take more than you need? Melatonin can be given to children, but you should always consult your doctor first and keep the dose less than 0.3 mg daily.

For adults, a dose of 0.1 to 0.3 mg before bedtime for insomnia is effective for many people, but you can gradually increase the dose up to 1 to 3 mg if needed. For jet lag, 0.5 to 5 mg one hour before arriving at your final destination can be helpful. Melatonin is available in both quick-release and sustained-release forms, and study results are mixed on which form works better, so you may need to experiment.

Cautionary Tales

Some people report having vivid dreams or nightmares when they take melatonin. It can also cause daytime drowsiness if you take too high a dose. Other side effects may include dizziness, headache, irritability, decreased libido, stomach

cramps, and breast enlargement in men. Doses between 1 and
5 mg have been known to cause seizures in children younger
than 15 years old. Women who are pregnant or breastfeeding
should not take melatonin because it can interfere with fertil-
ity. Melatonin may worsen symptoms of depression.

MSM

Methylsulfonylmethane (MSM) is a supplement form of sulfur, a naturally occurring mineral found in some plants, garlic,
asparagus, kale, wheat germ, eggs, fish, and legumes. MSM is
important for keeping your joints and connective tissues
healthy, and it also has been shown to slow down the nerve
signals that transmit pain messages, which thus reduces pain.

What Are the Benefits?

MSM is a popular supplement for treating the pain associated with arthritis and the symptoms of heartburn. Topical
forms of MSM are effective in treating skin conditions, including acne and rashes.

How Much Should I Take?

A common starting dose of MSM is 500 mg daily, and then
gradually increased to 1,000 mg and more, depending on the
condition you are treating. MSM is very well tolerated at
even high doses of 10 grams, but most people get relief from
their symptoms at levels between 4,000 to 8,000 mg daily (1
to 2 teaspoons). You should always drink lots of water when
taking MSM. For skin conditions, commercially available
MSM creams or gels can be applied one to three times daily.

Cautionary Tales

MSM appears to be safe, even at very high doses or when
taken along with conventional medications. However, you
should consult your doctor before taking large doses.

N-ACETYLCYSTEINE (NAC)

N-acetylcysteine is a form of the amino acid cysteine. One of its main functions is to help the body make glutathione, an important antioxidant that has a major role in supporting the immune system and eliminating toxins from the body. NAC also helps to make new cells to replace old, unhealthy cells, and plays a part in producing enzymes that protect the body from disease.

What Are the Benefits?

NAC has the ability to treat respiratory conditions, such as bronchitis, colds and flu, and pneumonia, because it can loosen mucus. NAC is especially helpful with colds and flu, as it can help prevent infection, reduce the symptoms once they occur, and reduce how long you suffer with the symptoms. Smokers can benefit from taking NAC because it can fight the free radicals produced by smoke. In another area of the body, NAC can help relieve symptoms of inflammatory bowel disease.

How Much Should I Take?

NAC is available in capsules and tablets. For cold and flu symptoms, as well as inflammatory bowel disease, the suggested adult dose is 600 mg twice daily. Children ages 6 to 12 may take one-quarter the dose and those ages 12 and older may take one-half the dose. NAC should be taken on an empty stomach. When taking NAC, it is recommended that you also take two to three times as much vitamin C, which helps keep the glutathione in a form that allows it to continue working as an antioxidant.

Cautionary Tales

Side effects associated with NAC do not occur often, but can include nausea, vomiting, constipation, and diarrhea. Rarely it causes rash, fever, drowsiness, or low blood pressure. If you experience some stomach upset when taking NAC on an empty stomach, take it with food.

OMEGA-3 FATTY ACIDS

Omega-3 essential fatty acids are a group of polyunsaturated fats that include eicosapentaenoic acid (EPA), docosahexaenoic acid (DHA), and alpha-linolenic acid (ALA), all of which play important roles in the body. All cells in the body need omega-3s to help keep their membranes flexible, which allows nutrients to enter the cells easily.

The omega-3s are found primarily in certain cold-water fish, including tuna, salmon, mackerel, and sardines. These sources offer EPA and DHA, which are the ingredients found in fish oil supplements. Other omega-3 sources include flaxseed, walnuts, hemp, and pumpkin seeds, and they offer ALA, the ingredient found in flaxseed and hemp seed supplements.

Experts say most people do not get enough omega-3s, and that it is important to maintain a healthy balance of omega-3 and omega-6 (another type of essential fatty acid) in the diet. One reason is that while omega-3s help reduce inflammation, most omega-6s promote it. Omega-6s are found in animal foods such as meat and poultry, and some vegetables oils, such as soybean and safflower.

Although fish oil supplements are a popular way to get omega-3 fatty acids, not everyone likes or wants to take fish oil. Flaxseed oil supplements provide ALA, which the body can use to make EPA and DHA. The conversion rate is not good, however, ranging from 5 to 25 percent. Therefore, to make enough EPA and DHA, you need to consume five to six times more ALA than if you took fish oil alone. One option is to take one tablespoon of flaxseed oil, which contains 8,000 mg of ALA.

A deficiency of omega-3s can lead to fatigue, poor memory, dry skin, heart problems, mood swings, and poor circulation. Some of these symptoms reflect the fact that omega-3s are highly concentrated in the brain.

What Are the Benefits?

It seems that new studies about the benefits of omega-3s are coming out all the time. Omega-3s have been shown to reduce inflammation, lower blood pressure, reduce cholesterol levels, relieve depression, help people who have ADHD, ease symptoms of arthritis, and improve symptoms of asthma, among other benefits.

How Much Should I Take?

How much fish oil you take should be based on the amount of EPA and DHA in the supplement and not on the total amount of fish oil. Supplements vary in the amounts of EPA and DHA that they contain, but a common amount in fish oil capsules is 180 mg (0.18 grams) of EPA and 120 mg (0.12 grams) of DHA. If you see a 1,000 mg capsule of fish oil, check out how much EPA and DHA it contains. For healthy adults, a suggested amount is 300 to 500 mg of EPA and DHA combined, plus an additional 800 to 1,100 mg of ALA.

Dosing can differ widely depending on the condition you are treating. Remember, a child's dose generally ranges from one-quarter (ages six to 12) to one-half (ages 12 and older) of an adult dose.

Cautionary Tales

Omega-3 supplements from fish oil may cause belching, flatulence, diarrhea, or a slightly fishy body odor. You can minimize or eliminate these symptoms if you take the supplement with food and if you start with a low dose and gradually increase it. When shopping for fish oil supplements, look for items that are marked as mercury-free or free of toxins. Such a statement is no guarantee of the supplement's purity, however. A recent study (February 2010) reported that eight of the top-selling omega-3 supplements were found to contain PCBs.

PROBIOTICS

Probiotics is a term for the "good bacteria" that normally live in your intestinal tract and that can be found in certain foods, such as yogurt, as well as nutritional supplements. Most often, the bacteria come from two groups: *Lactobacillus* and *Bifidobacterium,* each of which makes up a major part of the normal microflora in humans. Each group contains different species, and within each species, different varieties. A few probiotics are yeasts, such as *Saccharomyces boulardii.*

Ideally, good bacteria exist in a balance with harmful or "bad" bacteria in the intestinal tract. When the balance is in favor of the harmful bacteria, a variety of health complications can occur. Probiotic supplements can be taken to fight the negative effects of disease-causing organisms and restore the balance of intestinal bacteria.

What Are the Benefits?

Probiotics have been shown to be effective in treating diarrhea (especially diarrhea caused by rotavirus) and to help prevent and treat urinary tract infections and eczema (atopic dermatitis) in children. They also may be helpful in relieving symptoms of inflammatory bowel disease and ulcers.

How Much Should I Take?

Probiotics should be consumed daily to maintain both intestinal and overall health. Because many people do not eat enough foods that contain beneficial bacteria, probiotic supplements are recommended. A starting dose of 10 to 50 billion CFUs (colony-forming units, which is how probiotics are measured) is suggested for adults, with half that dose for children 12 and younger. Dosing is highly individual and also depends on whether you are treating a condition or maintaining health. When treating a gastrointestinal or allergy condition, for example, the suggested treatment may be 50 billion CFUs several times a day. Once symptoms begin to improve, you can gradually decrease the dose until you are taking a maintenance dose of about 10 to 50 billion CFUs.

Cautionary Tales

Probiotics may cause gas or stomach discomfort in some people, especially when they first start taking them, as the intestinal tract adjusts to the changing bacteria levels. This effect is temporary. Theoretically, taking very large doses of probiotics could cause infections that would require antibiotics to eliminate, but taking probiotics at recommended levels should be safe.

SAM-e

The supplement SAM-e (S-adenosylmethionine, also known as SAM) is a synthetic form of a compound that the body forms naturally from the amino acid methionine and the energy-producing molecule called adenosine triphosphate, or ATP. The fact that every cell in the body contains some SAM-e indicates just how important this substance is. In fact, it contributes to more than 100 different processes in the body. As we age, the body produces less and less SAM-e, so it is often used as a supplement to treat symptoms of different disorders that appear as we grow older.

What Are the Benefits?

Two of the most successful uses for SAM-e are in the treatment of osteoarthritis and depression. For osteoarthritis, SAM-e can protect the joints and promote the formation of cartilage. The supplement can also reduce inflammation and pain, which in turn allows patients to improve their mobility and range of motion. The success of SAM-e in the treatment of depression is attributed to its apparent ability to increase the availability of two neurotransmitters involved in mood, serotonin and dopamine. When compared with antidepressant medications, SAM-e has provided faster results and with few to no side effects.

How Much Should I Take?

SAM-e is available as capsules and tablets. A typical dose is 400 mg three times daily, but you can increase it as necessary up to 3,200 mg daily in divided doses. SAM-e can be safely taken with other natural antidepressants such as St. John's wort, as well as conventional antidepressants.

The best time to take SAM-e is two hours before or three hours after a meal, as the body absorbs it best on an empty stomach. If you experience heartburn or nausea, take it with lots of water. Avoid taking SAM-e late in the day because the supplement can cause a mild boost in energy and may cause insomnia. You can expect to notice benefits from SAM-e after about one week of treatment.

Although there are no proven or tested doses for SAM-e in children younger than 18, you can consult your physician about possible use for your child.

Cautionary Tales

SAM-e should not be used along with an MAO inhibitor. Always take a high-potency vitamin B complex supplement along with SAM-e, because as SAM-e breaks down in the body, it forms homocysteine, an amino acid that can cause heart problems and stroke if the levels reach high concentrations. The B vitamins can disarm homocysteine. A typical dose is 100 mg of a B complex once daily, regardless of your SAM-e dose.

If you have bipolar disorder, anxiety disorder, or another psychiatric condition, you should consult with your doctor before taking SAM-e. This supplement should not be taken by anyone who has Parkinson's disease. Side effects are not common, but if they do occur they can include nausea, rash, dry mouth, blood in the stool, thirst, increased urination, headache, hyperactivity, anxiety, and insomnia.

VITAMIN C

Vitamin C, also known as ascorbic acid, is probably the most well-known of all the vitamins among young and old alike. This is partly due to the media, which has associated vitamin C with orange juice and sunshine. This vitamin is critical for life, and because it is water-soluble, it needs to be replenished every day. Most people do not have a problem with that, as many popular foods contain healthy amounts of the vitamin, including bell peppers, cantaloupe, grapefruit, lemons, oranges, pineapple, raspberries, strawberries, tomatoes, and watermelon, as well as leafy green vegetables. In fact, vitamin C deficiency is very rare in the United States.

What Are the Benefits?

Vitamin C is a potent antioxidant, thus it helps protect the body against damaging free radicals and helps support the immune system. It also plays a key role in the health of the skin and gums, participates in the formation of collagen, a protein that makes up bones, tendons, teeth, and blood vessels, as well as protects against the development of cancer, cardiovascular diseases, and cataracts.

Most people think of fighting colds and flu with vitamin C, but many studies show that taking lots of vitamin C does little to help these viral infections. However, that certainly does not mean vitamin C isn't important. While you can take it for colds and flu, it also provides benefits for people who have asthma, anemia, and urinary tract infections, among other conditions.

How Much Should I Take?

The RDA for vitamin C is 75 mg for women, 90 mg for men, and lower amounts for children and adolescents, but most health professionals agree that these values are much too low. In fact, 500 to 1,000 mg is often suggested by experts. Since vitamin C is water-soluble, there is no fear of suffering any serious consequences of taking a higher dose. Some people take 10,000 mg or more without problems. However, high amounts of vitamin C can cause loose stools in some sensitive individuals. If you want to increase your intake of this vitamin, do is gradually, perhaps increasing your daily dose by 100 mg every three to four days until you notice symptoms, then reducing your dose accordingly.

Cautionary Tales

If you experience any stomach discomfort when taking vitamin C, you may want to take a buffered form, which usually combines the vitamin with magnesium, potassium, or calcium.

VITAMIN D

This "sunshine vitamin" is not really a vitamin at all, but a type of hormone. The body manufactures vitamin D when the skin is exposed to the sun's ultraviolet rays. Just 10 to 15 minutes of exposure to sunlight without sunscreen three times a week is believed by many experts to be enough for the body to make all the vitamin D that it needs. However, not all sunlight is the same: The closer you are to the equator, the more benefit you get from the sun's rays. Also, people who have darker skin need more sun exposure than lighter-skinned people.

Certain parts of the body are more efficient at making vitamin D, so make sure you expose your face, arms, legs, and back to the sun. Once you've gotten your dose of vitamin D sunshine, put on your sunscreen or go inside out of the sunlight.

Vitamin D is also available in some foods, including fortified milk and cereals, tuna, salmon, mackerel, liver, and egg yolks. Once you consume foods that contain vitamin D or your skin makes it, the kidneys and liver convert it into a hormone form that then provides the body with a variety of benefits.

What Are the Benefits?

Once the kidneys and liver do their job, the hormone form sends signals to the intestinal tract to increase the absorption of calcium and phosphorus, which is critical for strong, healthy bones. An increasing number of studies are showing that vitamin D is essential not only in maintaining bones and teeth, but also in fighting colds and flu, high cholesterol, and inflammatory bowel disease, and there is some evidence that it is helpful in depression, some cancers, and obesity. Researchers at Moores Cancer Center at the University of California, San Diego, for example, report that 600,000 cases of breast and colorectal cancers around the world could be prevented every year if people increased their intake of vitamin D and corrected their vitamin D deficiency.

How Much Should I Take?

If you can't get enough sunshine on a regular basis, and many people cannot, especially the elderly who may be housebound, it is important to take vitamin D supplements. The RDA for children and adults up to age 50 is 200 IU, then 400 IU up to age 70, and 600 IU thereafter. There is a growing consensus among health professionals that the requirement should be raised to 1,000 IU for everyone, but no official guidelines have yet been issued.

Data collected from the National Health and Nutrition Examination Survey (NHANES) found that 70 percent of children have abnormally low levels of vitamin D. Therefore parents should make sure their children get an adequate amount of sunshine and supplemental vitamin D.

Cautionary Tales

A vitamin D deficiency is associated with the development of rickets in children (soft bones that become malformed) and osteoporosis in adults. Deficiencies have also been linked with high blood pressure, depression, and heart disease. Although taking more than the RDA for vitamin D is considered safe, taking excessively high amounts can cause abdominal cramps, nausea, nervousness, and weakness. Children should not take more than 2,000 IU daily and adults should not exceed 10,000 IU daily.

VITAMIN E

Did you know that there are eight different members of the vitamin E family? If you have ever gone shopping for vitamin E supplements, you may have noticed two different types— tocopherol and tocotrienol—and each of these types come in four varieties: alpha-, beta-, gamma-, and delta- compounds. Of the eight, alpha-tocopherol is the most common and the one that is the most useful and active in the body.

Vitamin E is available in some foods, including wheat germ oil, almonds, hazelnuts, safflower oil, sunflower seeds, and peanut butter, and in supplements. As an antioxidant, this fat-soluble vitamin fights free radicals to help prevent disease. It is also involved in immune system function, metabolism, and in preventing platelets from sticking together and forming blood clots.

What Are the Benefits?

It is important to get enough vitamin E because of its antioxidant activities, and especially because it is a heart-friendly vitamin. Research shows that vitamin E can reduce the development of plaque in the arteries and thus prevent the formation of blood clots, which can lead to a heart attack or stroke.

Another benefit of vitamin E is its ability to ease skin conditions, including eczema, psoriasis, and irritations. It is also effective in the treatment of vaginitis, both as an antioxidant against the various organisms that can cause this condition, and in soothing and healing.

How Much Should I Take?

The RDA for vitamin E is 4 to 11 mg (6–16.4 IU) from birth up to age 13, and then 15 mg (22.4 IU) thereafter. Many experts believe these values are much too low. Most supplements contain more than 100 IU per dose.

When purchasing vitamin E, either in a multivitamin or alone, you may see the amount given in mg or IU. Vitamin E content of foods and supplements is listed on labels in IUs, which is a measure of biological activity rather than quantity. Supplements of vitamin E usually provide only alpha-tocopherol, although there are some "mixed" vitamin E supplements on the market. Synthetically produced alpha-tocopherol is only about half as active as the same amount (by weight in mg) of natural alpha-tocopherol. This means that you need approximately 50 percent more IU of synthetic alpha-tocopherol from supplements and fortified foods to obtain the same amount of the nutrient as from the natural form.

If you need to translate the mgs to IUs or vice versa on a supplement, here are the conversion formulas:

- To convert from mg to IU: 1 mg of alpha-tocopherol is equal to 1.49 IU of the natural form or 2.22 IU of the synthetic form
- To convert from IU to mg: 1 IU of alpha-tocopherol is equal to 0.67 of the natural form or 0.45 mg of the synthetic form

Cautionary Tales

Vitamin E deficiency is rare, and obvious symptoms do not occur in healthy people who get little vitamin E from their diets. Vitamin E is fat soluble and thus the digestive tract requires fat to absorb it. People most likely to become vitamin E deficient are those who have a disorder that impairs their ability to absorb fat. Symptoms of deficiency include peripheral neuropathy, retinopathy, ataxia (incoordination and unsteadiness), and an impaired immune system.

ZINC

Zinc is a trace mineral that is found primarily in the muscles. The rest of this critical nutrient resides in the skin, bones, eyes, testes, prostate, and kidneys. Among its key functions are assisting in growth, sexual maturation, balancing blood sugar levels, regulating genetic activity, and balancing carbohydrate metabolism. Zinc is also involved with more than one hundred enzymes, including those that impact protein synthesis, bone development, thyroid function, and tissue growth and repair.

The richest food sources of zinc include almonds, dried beans, fortified cereals, milk, oatmeal, oysters, peas, seeds, walnuts, and yogurt. The RDA for zinc ranges from 3 mg for children ages 7 months to 8 to 11 mg for adults.

What Are the Benefits?

Zinc is an antioxidant and is well-known for its ability to boost the immune system and help fight common infections, such as cold and flu, and other infections that impact the respiratory tract. Studies also show zinc to be effective in treating acne. Zinc may help prevent hormone imbalances that can result in acne outbreaks, and it also is involved in protein synthesis and collagen formation, which are essential for healthy skin and normalizing production of skin oils.

How Much Should I Take?

Zinc supplements come in several forms, including zinc glycerate, zinc picolinate, zinc citrate, zinc acetate, and zinc sulfate. The first four forms are more readily absorbed by the body, while zinc sulfate is the least easily absorbed and can cause stomach upset. If you are treating a cold, you might try zinc lozenges, which should be used according to package directions.

Typical doses of zinc supplements for treating specific symptoms are less than 40 mg daily, because more than that can impair copper absorption. In some cases, as when treating acne, you may take higher doses of zinc for a limited amount of time (see "Acne"). In such cases, talk to your physician about taking additional copper to maintain the proper balance of zinc and copper.

Cautionary Tales

Zinc deficiency is not common in the United States. However, among certain groups of people, low levels of zinc may occur, including individuals who have digestive disorders (e.g., ulcerative colitis, Crohn's disease), vegetarians, pregnant and breastfeeding women, alcoholics, and people who have sickle cell disease. Symptoms include loss of appetite and impaired immune function. Prolonged use of diuretics can increase the amount of zinc you excrete by up to 60 percent, so you should monitor your zinc intake if you use these medications.

HERBAL SUPPLEMENTS

ALOE VERA

Aloe vera has been used for thousands of years to treat various conditions, and today it is one of the most commonly used herbs in the United States. The plant is available in more than 300 species, but only a few are used for healing. The leaves of this fleshy plant contain a gel that is useful for various ailments. The outer layer of the leaves also contain a bitter, yellow liquid known as aloe latex. This substance used to be used to treat constipation, but it is no longer recommended because the latex causes severe side effects.

What Are the Benefits?

Although aloe is 99 percent water, the gel also contains substances called glycoproteins and polysaccharides. Glycoproteins have the ability to stop pain and inflammation, while polysaccharides can help skin repair. Both substances are also believed to help stimulate the immune system.

Perhaps you have an aloe plant in your kitchen, where it is within easy reach if you or a family member suffers a burn or cut. But aloe is also effective for treatment of hemorrhoids and skin conditions such as eczema, psoriasis, acne, athlete's foot, and sunburn. Aloe vera juice can be used to treat heartburn, ulcers, and other gastrointestinal problems.

How Much Should I Take?

If you have an aloe plant at home, you can simply break off a leaf and split it open to get the healing gel for treating a skin condition. Aloe gel is also available in ointments, lotions, and creams. Aloe in any of these forms is safe for both children and adults and can be applied to the skin's surface several times a day.

Aloe vera juice (not the gel) can be taken to relieve symptoms of heartburn and GERD. A typical dose is ¼ cup of aloe vera juice 10 minutes before each meal. The juice soothes the mucous membranes and also helps to heal the lower esophageal sphincter, the one-way valve at the bottom of the esophagus where the acid from the stomach passes through up into the throat.

Cautionary Tales

Aloe gel is considered safe when applied to the skin, but do not apply it to open or deep wounds. If you develop a rash when using aloe gel, stop using it. If you want to use aloe juice, talk to your doctor before you do if you are taking glyburide to treat type 2 diabetes, because the combination may cause your blood sugar level to fall too low. Aloe also should not be taken if you use diuretics or digoxin (a medication used to treat irregular heart rhythms and congestive heart failure). Topical aloe is safe for pregnant and breastfeeding women, but they should not use aloe juice.

BUTTERBUR

The shrub called butterbur gets its name from the fact that in the days before refrigeration, people used to wrap butter in the plant's large, supple leaves. Today, butterbur *(Petasites hybridus)* is much better known for its ability to relieve symptoms of several common ailments. Its active ingredients are sesquiterpenes, including petasin and isopetasin.

What Are the Benefits?

Butterbur has anti-inflammatory properties and an ability to relax blood vessel walls. These factors make it a good candidate for treating migraine. Studies show that people who took butterbur were able to significantly reduce the number of migraine attacks.

If you suffer with allergic rhinitis, butterbur may help relieve your symptoms. Several small studies have shown butterbur to be as effective as cetirizine (Zyrtec) in relieving symptoms such as stuffy nose and itchy eyes, but without the drowsiness the medication can cause. Butterbur is also used to treat asthma and bronchitis, as there is evidence that it can reduce mucus production.

How Much Should I Take?

When shopping for butterbur supplements, look for those that are free of pyrrolizidine alkaloids (PAs), a naturally occurring substance that can cause liver damage. Butterbur extracts are typically standardized to contain a minimum of 7.5 mg of petasin and isopetasin. A typical adult dose of butterbur is 50 to 100 mg twice daily with meals. Children ages six to 12 years may take one-quarter to one-half the adult dose, while those older than 12 years may take one-half to the full adult dose.

Cautionary Tales

It has not been determined whether taking butterbur for longer than 12 to 16 weeks is safe. Pregnant and breastfeeding women should not take butterbur. If you are allergic to ragweed, marigolds, or daisies, you may want to avoid butterbur, as it may cause an allergic reaction. Other side effects are uncommon, but can include stomach upset, headache, and drowsiness.

CAPSAICIN

Chili peppers (cayenne peppers) are the source of capsaicin, an alkaloid that can bring tears to your eyes and a flush to your skin. Capsaicin is the key to the chili pepper's healing powers as well, and many cultures have taken advantage of those properties over the centuries. The Maya of Central America used cayenne peppers to fight infections, and the Aztecs utilized the herb to treat toothaches.

Modern science has confirmed that capsaicin has pain-relieving powers, which it achieves by depleting the nerve endings of a chemical neurotransmitter that is responsible for sending pain signals to the brain. Capsaicin also enhances blood flow and has been credited with antibacterial abilities. Although it seems logical to think that eating chili peppers would cause ulcers and stomach distress, studies actually show that lab animals fed high doses of aspirin did not develop ulcers when they were also given capsaicin.

What Are the Benefits?

Several studies have shown that this chili pepper compound is effective in reducing the pain of both shingles and postherpetic neuralgia, a condition that develops in some individuals once the rash from shingles has disappeared. Postherpetic neuralgia causes the skin to remain painful and hypersensitive for months to years once shingles has disappeared.

Capsaicin is also used to relieve the pain associated with arthritis, backache, diabetic neuropathy, and sprains. Some cancer patients with postsurgical pain have also experienced relief when using capsaicin.

How Much Should I Take?

Capsaicin is available as a lotion, cream, gel, liquid, and pads that can be applied to the skin. Strengths vary from 0.025 percent to 0.075 percent, and the topical can be applied three to four times daily.

Capsaicin causes a burning, stinging, or warm sensation when it is applied to the skin. This is a normal reaction and usually goes away after the first few days of use. It is necessary to keep using capsaicin in order to keep enjoying pain relief. It typically takes several days before you will notice significant relief in symptoms.

Cautionary Tales

Never apply capsaicin to broken skin. To avoid getting the substance into your eyes or other sensitive body parts, always wear gloves when applying capsaicin, and wash your hands with soap and water after using it.

CHAMOMILE

Chamomile is one of the world's most well-known medicinal herbs. Of the two species of chamomile, the German variety *(Matricaria recutita)* is used more often in the United States and has been studied more extensively than the Roman variety *(Chamaemelum nobile)*. German chamomile is a member of the daisy family, and its flowers are used to make the remedies.

Chamomile has been used since ancient times. The Egyptians valued it as a remedy for chills and fever, and people during medieval times used it for nervous stomach and to dissolve gallstones. Modern research has revealed that chamomile contains flavonoids (including one called apigenin), an essential oil, and many more compounds, including chamazulene and alpha-bisabolol. Overall, chamomile has been credited with anti-inflammatory, antibacterial, antifungal, antiseptic, and antispasmodic properties.

What Are the Benefits?

Perhaps you've treated yourself to a cup of chamomile tea when you've had trouble falling asleep. In fact, treating insomnia is one of the main reasons people use chamomile. Chamomile tea has also been used for centuries to relieve symptoms of colic. You may want to treat yourself to a cup of chamomile tea while treating your colicky infant, as chamomile is also used to calm the nervous system. Chamomile can also provide relief for strep throat, bloating, indigestion, and mouth and gum irritation.

How Much Should I Take?

Chamomile is available as a tea and in capsules, tablets, liquid extract, and tincture. Common dosages include 1 to 4 cups daily of tea (except for colic), 400 to 1,600 mg daily in capsules and tablets, 1 to 4 mL taken three times daily of the liquid extract, and 15 mL taken three to four times daily of the tincture.

Cautionary Tales

Do not use chamomile if you are allergic to ragweed, asters, mums, or other plants in the Asteraceae family. Side effects of chamomile may include rash or shortness of breath. Chamomile should not be used during pregnancy because there is a possibility it may stimulate the uterus.

CHASTEBERRY

The chasteberry tree *(Vitex agnus castsus)* grows in southern Europe and the Mediterranean area and provides us with a red-black berry and leaves that are rich in flavonoids and other active ingredients, including casticin, kaempferol, agnuside, and isovitexin, among others. The flowers and leaves contain progesterone, testosterone, and other hormones, but not estrogen. The berry is the part usually used for healing remedies.

What Are the Benefits?

Chasteberry is a popular herbal remedy for symptoms of PMS. Symptoms of PMS are usually caused by low progesterone levels in relation to estrogen, thus taking chasteberry can provide some relief. In one study, 77 percent of women suffering with PMS who took chasteberry experienced relief with bloating, irritability, depression, digestive problems, breast tenderness, skin problems, and weight gain.

How Much Should I Take?

Chasteberry is available as a tincture, an extract, a tea, or in capsules. The usual dosage is 200 mg of the berry, with a standardized amount (0.5%) of the active ingredient agnuside. If you choose the tincture of extracts, mix 10 to 30 drops in water or juice and take the dose three times daily. Chasteberry tea is made from 1 teaspoon of ripe berries added to 8 ounces of boiling water. Steep the berries for 10 to 15 minutes and drink one cup three times daily.

Cautionary Tales

Chasteberry may affect your hormone levels, so if you are pregnant, taking birth control pills, or have a hormone-related condition, do not take this herb. Some women experience mild dizziness, diarrhea, headache, rash, or gastrointestinal discomfort when using chasteberry.

CINNAMON

Cinnamon (*Cinnamomum zeylanicum, C. cassia*) is one of the oldest spices and healing remedies known to man. It is derived from the bark of the cinnamon tree, which grows in India, Sri Lanka, Indonesia, Brazil, Egypt, and Vietnam. Of the two varieties of cinnamon, Chinese (or cassia) and Ceylon, the latter is slightly sweeter, more refined, and more difficult to find.

The bark, which is dried and ground into a powder, contains three active components in its essential oils: cinnamaldehyde, cinnamyl acetate, and cinnamyl alcohol, plus various other substances. These three components are believed to be the source of cinnamon's healing abilities.

What Are the Benefits?

Traditionally, cinnamon has been used to treat colds, nausea, diarrhea, and painful menstruation, as well as diabetes and indigestion. Scientific studies have found that cinnamon can benefit people who have type 2 diabetes. The spice may reduce fasting blood glucose, triglycerides, "bad" cholesterol (low-density lipoprotein, or LDL), and total cholesterol. Cinnamon is also useful in treating sore and strep throat and has shown some promise as an antifungal agent, which makes it a possible remedy for yeast infections.

How Much Should I Take?

Research indicates that as little as 1 gram per day (¼ to ½ teaspoon) of cinnamon can reduce blood glucose by 20 percent, along with cholesterol and triglycerides. In some studies, patients with diabetes have taken from 1 to 6 grams in pill form daily. It is best to start low and gradually increase the amount of cinnamon you take while monitoring its impact on your blood glucose levels.

Cinnamon tea is often suggested as the best way to treat yeast infections. To prepare the tea, add 8 to 10 sticks of cinnamon to 4 cups of boiling water and let them simmer for 5 minutes. Remove the pot from the heat and let the cinnamon steep for about 45 minutes. Drink 1 to 2 cups daily.

Cautionary Tales

If you have diabetes and are taking medication for the disease, do not take cinnamon until you talk to your doctor. Nor should you begin taking cinnamon and stop taking your diabetes medication without consulting your physician. Cinnamon is safe when taken in the recommended amounts. It is possibly unsafe if taken in large amounts for long periods of time, in that it may cause or worsen liver disease in sensitive individuals. Women who are pregnant or breastfeeding should not take cinnamon supplements.

CRANBERRY

Cranberries (*Vaccinium macrocarpon*) were a favorite among the Native Americans, who used them to treat bladder and kidney diseases. Little did the settlers realize that the natives would be introducing them to a fruit that not only would be a traditional Thanksgiving Day food, but an effective remedy as well.

Cranberries are related to blueberries, huckleberries, and buckberries, and are found mainly in North America. The fruit are high in antioxidants, many of which are substances called proanthocyanidins. Antioxidants fight cell-damaging molecules called free radicals, which are associated with disease and aging. Cranberries are also an excellent source of vitamin C, another antioxidant.

What Are the Benefits?

Cranberries are best known as a preventive treatment for urinary tract infections. This fruit has the ability to prevent the bacteria that cause these infections to attach to the walls of the urinary tract. Studies show that cranberry supplements or juice can prevent urinary tract infections, and that the supplements are more effective than the juice. Research also indicates that cranberries are more effective at preventing rather than treating urinary tract infections, although they do offer some benefit. Cranberries are also helpful in the treatment of ulcers, and there is some suggestion that they may help prevent buildup of plaque in the arteries and assist in preventing bacteria from sticking to gums and around the teeth.

How Much Should I Take?

Cranberries are available fresh or frozen and as juice and concentrate, or as a supplement in capsule and tablet form. If you use the juice, look for pure cranberry juice (no sugar added), or one that has a little sugar as possible. To help prevent urinary tract infections, the suggested dose for adults is 3 or more ounces of pure cranberry juice daily, or 300 to 400 mg, six capsules or tablets daily in divided doses. Children may take one-quarter to one-half the adult dose. If your child has a urinary tract infection, he or she should also see a physician for treatment.

Cautionary Tales

Cranberry is considered safe with no serious side effects, even for pregnant and breastfeeding women. Because cranberry contains high levels of oxalate, chemicals that can increase the risk of kidney stones, talk to your doctor about taking cranberry juice or supplement if you have had kidney stones. Cranberry may interfere with the effects of the blood-thinning drug warfarin.

DANDELION

For some people, the dandelion *(Taraxacum officinale)* is a weed, but for others, it is an effective remedy. For centuries, dandelion leaves have been used medicinally as a diuretic, while the roots have acted as a blood purifier that can stimulate the liver and kidneys to remove toxins from the blood. The flowers are a good source of antioxidants.

Dandelion also is a mild laxative and improves digestion and the appetite. The herb contains various nutrients, including high levels of potassium as well as iron, zinc, calcium, B vitamins, and vitamins A, C, and D. And as a bonus, the leaves and flowers have been enjoyed in various recipes. Perhaps this *dents de lion,* or lion's tooth, as the French call this plant, is not a weed after all!

What Are the Benefits?

Unlike conventional diuretics, dandelion does not cause a loss of potassium because it is rich in this nutrient. Thus dandelion is helpful in relieving water retention and bloating associated with premenstrual syndrome. Its high potassium content also aids in alleviating muscle spasms and leg cramps. The herb is also helpful in treating anemia due to deficiencies of folic acid, iron and vitamin B_{12}.

Dandelion root is a mild bitter, and bitters help increase the secretion of digestive juices and stimulates production of bile. Increased bile relieves constipation and also helps with hemorrhoids.

How Much Should I Take?

Dandelion is available as a tablet, tea, or tincture. Children can take this remedy; all you have to do is adjust the recommended adult dose to account for the child's weight. If your child weighs 50 pounds, the suggested dose of dandelion would be one-third of the adult dosage; at 100 pounds, two-thirds is recommended.

Adult doses are as follows: For tea made from the dried leaf, use 1 to 2 teaspoons steeped in hot water for 5 to 10 minutes. Drink up to 3 cups daily. If you choose dried root, use ½ to 2 teaspoons in boiling water for 5 to 10 minutes. Drink up to 3 cups daily. To use the standardized powdered extract leaf or root, take 500 mg one to three times daily. The leaf tincture (30 percent alcohol) or root tincture (45 percent alcohol) can be taken at 100 to 150 drops, three times daily.

Cautionary Tales

If you have an allergy to plants related to dandelion, such as chamomile and yarrow, use dandelion with caution. Dandelion should not be used if you are taking antibiotics, especially ciprofloxacin, ofloxacin, and others in this group, because the herb may prevent the drugs from effectively fighting infections.

DEVIL'S CLAW

Devil's claw *(Harpagophytum procumbens)* is a South African herb that has an unusual fruit, which is covered with claw-like structures. The medicinal part of the herb is the root, which has been traditionally used to treat arthritis, fever, malaria, sore muscles, and to clear toxins from the blood. Scientific studies show that the herb contains a chemical called harpagoside, which has anti-inflammatory properties.

What Are the Benefits?

Devil's claw is currently used as an anti-inflammatory and pain reliever for joint pain, back pain, and headache. In one study, for example, devil's claw relieved the pain associated with osteoarthritis as effectively as a popular painkilling drug. Another study found devil's claw to significantly reduce pain associated with rheumatic disorders and to improve quality of life in those patients.

How Much Should I Take?

Suggested doses of devil's claw include 0.2 to 0.25 mL of the liquid extract three times daily or, with tablets, 600 to 1,200 mg of extract standardized to contain 50 to 100 mg of harpagoside, taken three times daily. This herb generally is not given to children.

Cautionary Tales

Devil's claw is generally well tolerated. Possible side effects include headache, ringing in the ears, low blood pressure, abnormal heart rhythms, or gastrointestinal upset. If you are taking blood thinners (e.g., warfarin) or have stomach ulcers, talk to your doctor before taking devil's claw. Because devil's claw theoretically may lower blood sugar levels, be cautious if you have diabetes as the herb may cause your levels to go too low.

ECHINACEA

Echinacea *(Echinacea purpurea)* is one of the most popular and commonly used herbs in the United States. It has a long tradition in America, as it was used extensively by the Great Plains Indian tribes to treat snakebites, wounds, coughs, sore throat, respiratory problems, digestive disorders, and tooth- aches, among other uses. Today, echinacea continues to be used for many of these same ailments.

Echinacea contains several ingredients, including glyco- proteins, flavonoids, caffeic acid derivatives, and alkylamides, which are believed to be responsible for its ability to boost function of the immune system to fight infections. Studies indicate that the herb has antiviral properties and promotes activity of infection-fighting white blood cells.

What Are the Benefits?

Echinacea's effect on the immune system enables it to help immune system cells destroy invading organisms, including those that cause bronchitis, colds, flu, ear infections, and strep throat. Research indicates that echinacea may reduce inflammation, strengthen blood vessels, and even help pre- vent sun damage to the skin.

How Much Should I Take?

Typical dosages of echinacea include up to nine 300- to 400-mg capsules taken throughout the day, or up to 60 drops of tincture taken three times daily. Echinacea should be taken for no longer than two weeks, followed by one week without the herb, then back to two weeks of dosing. Children may take echinacea, but at a reduced dose. For children who weigh 50 pounds, one-third the adult dose is typical; those who weigh 100 pounds may take two-thirds the dose.

Cautionary Tales

Echinacea is not recommended for people who have diabetes, multiple sclerosis, HIV, or an autoimmune condition. If you are allergic to other members of the daisy family, it is possible you will be allergic to echinacea as well. Side effects are not common and may include diarrhea, dry mouth, fever, heartburn, and nausea.

FEVERFEW

The name "feverfew" reveals the original use of this herb from ancient times. to "chase away fever," but it was also used to treat headache and menstrual complaints. Today, feverfew *(Tanacetum parthenium)* is perhaps best known as a treatment for migraine, but it did not gain much attention for this use until the mid-1970s, when a Welsh doctor's wife ate fresh feverfew leaves and got relief from her chronic migraines.

The active ingredient in feverfew is believed to be parthenolide, which has the ability to relieve smooth muscle spasms and prevent the constriction of blood vessels in the brain. Parthenolide also inhibits the activity of substances that promote inflammation, and it is possible that it may also have an impact on cancer growth, although this has not been determined.

What Are the Benefits?

Migraine relief remains the main reason why people take feverfew. Studies show that it can reduce the frequency of migraines by more than 50 percent. In addition, the herb's anti-inflammatory properties have also been helpful in relieving symptoms of arthritis and other inflammatory conditions.

How Much Should I Take?

Feverfew is available in capsules, tablets, and extracts made from dried leaves. You can also buy dried leaves to make tea. For migraines, the suggested dosage for adults is 100 to 300 mg up to four times daily, using the standardized form containing 0.2 to 0.4 parthenolides. For preventing migraine, you can take the carbon dioxide extracted form: 6.25 mg three times daily for up to 16 weeks.

For arthritis and other inflammatory conditions, the suggested dose is 60 to 120 drops of fluid extract twice daily. To make feverfew tea, steep one teaspoon of the dried leaves in 5 to 8 ounces of water and boil for 5 to 10 minutes. Strain the leaves and drink as much tea as you desire per day.

This herb should not be given to children younger than two years of age. In older children, the dose is a percentage that is calculated based on an average of 150 pound adult. Therefore, a 50 pound child could take one-third the adult dose; a 100 pound child could take two-thirds of the dose.

Cautionary Tales

Although feverfew leaves can be chewed, this can cause mouth and stomach irritation and is discouraged. Side effects from other forms of feverfew may include abdominal pain, indigestion, diarrhea, nausea, vomiting, and nervousness. Allergic reactions are rare, though if you are allergic to ragweed, yarrow, or chamomile, you should not take feverfew. If you have a bleeding disorder or take blood-thinning medications, do not take feverfew until you consult your healthcare provider. Pregnant and breastfeeding women should not take feverfew.

If you have been using feverfew for more than one week, do not suddenly stop taking it, as you may experience withdrawal symptoms, such as rebound headache, fatigue, muscle stiffness, and joint pain. Taper off the remedy gradually by reducing your dosage by a quarter each day.

GARLIC

You may love it on your pizza and add it to your pasta sauce, but garlic is also a healing herb. Use of garlic as both food and medicine goes back to the days of the pharaohs in Egypt. Garlic was taken to fight off the plague in medieval Europe and by soldiers during World Wars I and II to prevent gangrene.

Garlic is a natural healer because it is rich in antioxidants, making it a powerful enemy of cell-damaging free radicals. Today garlic is used to prevent and treat a wide variety of ailments, as you'll see below.

The active ingredient in garlic is alliin, an odorless sulfur-containing chemical. When you crush or chew fresh garlic, alliin is converted into another compound called allicin. This is the substance that appears to be one of the main active ingredients that gives garlic both its characteristic fragrance and its healing powers. Because allicin is not absorbed effectively by the body, aged garlic is fermented to break allicin down to substances that the body can use easily.

What Are the Benefits?

Numerous studies show that garlic can not only help prevent the buildup of cholesterol in blood vessels but also treat high cholesterol. Garlic is taken to reduce high blood pressure and to boost the immune system to assist in fighting allergies, athlete's foot, bronchitis, cold and flu, diarrhea, ear infections, and vaginitis. There are also studies looking at the benefits of garlic in the fight against cancer, but more research needs to be done in this area.

How Much Should I Take?

Fresh garlic is a wonderful natural medicine, but you may prefer to get yours in a supplement. Garlic supplements are made from whole fresh garlic, dried or freeze-dried garlic, garlic oil, and aged garlic extracts, available in capsules and tablets. Aged garlic products are made by fermenting garlic. If possible, use standardized aged garlic supplements, as they are better absorbed and utilized by the body.

Standard dosages of garlic for adults include 2 to 4 grams daily of fresh, minced garlic (each clove is about 1 gram), 600 to 1,200 mg daily of aged garlic extract, or 200 mg, two to three times daily, of freeze-dried garlic standardized to 1.3% alliin or 0.6% allicin. Garlic oil can also be used: 0.03 to 0.12 mL three times daily is suggested. For children, you may give one-quarter the adult dose to children ages six to 12 and one-half the adult dose for children 12 to 17.

Cautionary Tales

Garlic is considered to be a very safe herb. However, some people experience bloating, upset stomach, bad breath, and body odor when using garlic. In rare cases, garlic can cause headache, fatigue, muscle aches, dizziness, and an allergic reaction or rash (usually from touching fresh garlic).

Garlic has the ability to thin the blood, so talk to your doctor before using garlic if you are taking blood thinning medication, such as warfarin. The combination could increase the risk of bleeding.

GINGER

The tropical plant known as ginger *(Zingiber officinale)* is one of the most popular herbs in the world. The underground stem (rhizome) is used as a spice and for medicinal purposes. Since ancient times, those healing purposes have included stomachaches, diarrhea, arthritis, heart conditions, and nausea. The components in ginger that are believed to be responsible for these benefits include volatile oils and phenol compounds, such as gingerols and shogaols.

What Are the Benefits?

Ginger may be best known for its ability to help prevent and treat nausea, whether it is associated with PMS, pregnancy, the flu, migraine, or another ailment. But ginger is also useful in relieving symptoms of colic and diarrhea, and it is a flavor that many children like. In fact, ginger is one of the few herbal remedies you can enjoy candied. If your child tends to get motion sickness, he or she can chew on candied ginger while traveling to help relieve any nauseous feelings.

How Much Should I Take?

Ginger supplements are made from fresh or dried ginger root or from steam distillation of the oil found in the root. Extracts, tinctures, capsules, and oils are readily available. If you prefer to make ginger tea, you can buy fresh ginger root.

For diarrhea, gas, or nausea, a suggested dose is 2 to 4 grams of fresh root daily or 30 to 90 drops of liquid extract daily. An alternative is 75 to 2,000 mg in divided doses, standardized to contain 4 percent volatile oils or 5 percent 6-gingerol or 6-shogaol. Take ginger supplements with food. To make ginger tea, steep 2 tablespoons of freshly shredded ginger in boiling water for 5 to 10 minutes. Drink two to three cups daily.

For children older than two years old, ginger can relieve diarrhea, nausea, digestive cramping, and headache. Adjust the adult dose as follows: one-third the adult dose for children who weigh 50 pounds, and two-thirds the dose for those weighing 100 pounds.

Cautionary Tales

Ginger typically does not cause side effects, but if you take more than suggested amounts, you may experience mild heartburn, irritation of the mouth, and diarrhea. If you have gallstones, talk to your doctor before taking ginger. Do not take ginger if you have a bleeding disorder or if you are taking blood-thinning medications.

GINKGO

The ginkgo tree *(Ginkgo biloba)* is one of the oldest living tree species, and its leaves have been studied extensively for their healing powers. In traditional medicine, ginkgo has been used to treat circulatory disorders and to boost memory, and scientific studies have found some evidence to support these uses. Some of these studies have uncovered ginkgo's antioxidant properties, which are attributed to two types of chemicals found in the leaves, flavonoids and terpenoids. Flavonoids have been found to protect the nerves, heart muscle, and retina from free-radical damage. Terpenoids (e.g., ginkgolides) help improve blood flow by dilating blood vessels.

What Are the Benefits?

Ginkgo's antioxidant powers help maintain the health of blood vessels, which in turn improves blood flow to the brain and other parts of the body. The herb is especially useful in improving microcirculation in the capillaries, and this ability has led to ginkgo being used to treat erectile dysfunction. Ginkgo also has anti-inflammatory abilities, and studies indicate that it is helpful in relieving symptoms of asthma because it may interfere with the protein in the blood that causes spasms of the airways.

Studies of ginkgo's ability to improve memory and other cognitive functions and to possibly delay the symptoms of Alzheimer's disease and other dementias have yielded conflicting results. A large study conducted at the University of Pittsburgh and published in late 2009 found that ginkgo was no better than placebo in preventing dementia or Alzheimer's, while other studies have shown some benefit.

How Much Should I Take?

Ginkgo supplements are available in capsules, tablets, and liquid extracts, and as dried leaves for tea. The suggested adult dose is 120 mg daily in divided doses standardized to contain 24 to 32% flavonoids (may appear as flavones glycosides or heterosides on the label) and 6 to 12% terpenoids (triterpene lactones). Doses for children are based on body weight: one-third of the adult dose for children who weigh 50 pounds, two-thirds for those who weigh 100 pounds. However, consult your doctor before giving ginkgo to a child.

Cautionary Tales

Ginkgo seldom causes side effects, but they may include headache, rash, dizziness, and gastrointestinal upset. The herb may cause bleeding in people who are taking blood-thinning drugs or who have a bleeding disorder. Ginkgo also should not be used if you are pregnant or breastfeeding or if you have epilepsy. Because ginkgo may lower blood pressure, talk to your doctor before taking ginkgo if you are taking blood pressure medication.

GINSENG

The word "ginseng" is used to refer to the American *(Panax quinquefolius)* and the Korean or Asian ginseng *(Panax ginseng)*. (Siberian ginseng is not the same, has different effects, and is in a different family.) Both American and Asian ginseng contain ginsenosides, substances that are credited with providing ginseng with its healing abilities.

What Are the Benefits?

Among ginseng's many benefits is its role as an adaptogen, which means it can help the body cope with stress. Ginseng is an antioxidant and thus helps protect the body against damaging free radicals. Studies have also shown that ginseng can boost the immune system, reduce risk of cancer, and improve mental functioning. It has proven especially useful in lowering blood sugar levels in people who have type 2 diabetes, and some men use it to treat erectile dysfunction.

How Much Should I Take?

Ginseng is available in both water and alcohol liquid extracts, and in powders, tablets, and capsules. The suggested dose for adults is 100 to 200 mg, one to three times daily, of extract standardized to contain 4 to 5 percent ginsenosides. You can also take ¼ to ½ teaspoon of fluid extract (1:1) one to three times daily, or 1 to 2 teaspoons of tincture (1:5) one to three times daily. Ginseng should be taken with food.

Regardless of which ginseng form you take, do not use it for more than two to three weeks continuously. Take a one-week break from ginseng before resuming it.

Cautionary Tales

Side effects are not common, but they can include high blood pressure, insomnia, anxiety, diarrhea, euphoria, vomiting, headache, nosebleed, vaginal bleeding, or breast pain. Do not take ginseng if you are pregnant or breastfeeding. Ginseng may increase the effects of medications used to treat psychiatric disorders such as bipolar disorder and those taken for attention deficit hyperactivity disorder.

GOLDENSEAL

Goldenseal is one of the best-selling herbal remedies in the United States. The herb used to grow mainly in the wild, but its popularity caused it to be overharvested, and so today much of goldenseal is grown on farms.

Goldenseal is often found in combination remedies with echinacea because it is widely believed that goldenseal enhances the benefits of echinacea, even though this has not been proven scientifically.

What Are the Benefits?

Research indicates that goldenseal contains a substance called berberine, which has anti-inflammatory and antibacterial properties. Berberine has also killed other germs in test tubes, such as candida (yeast) infections and various parasites. Berberine may also help make white blood cells more effective at fighting infections.

Goldenseal appears to contain only a small amount of berberine, yet this has not stopped many people from taking the supplement for a variety of ailments, including colds and flu, bronchitis, and ear infections. It is also used in mouthwashes for sore throats and canker sores.

One reported "benefit" of goldenseal is that taking the herb can help mask a positive test for illegal drugs. Studies have shown that this is not true.

How Much Should I Take?

The typical dose of goldenseal depends on the form. Goldenseal is available as tablets and capsules (containing powdered root) and liquid extracts. For dried root in tablets or capsules, 500 to 1,000 mg three times daily is standard. For the liquid extract, take ½ to 1 teaspoon three times daily. Children who weigh 50 pounds can take one-third the adult dose; those weighing 100 pounds can be given two-thirds the dose.

Cautionary Tales

If you have a known allergy or hypersensitivity to goldenseal or any of its constituents, such as berberine or hydrastine, you should not use this herb. Side effects are not common and may include nausea, vomiting, or numbness in the arms or legs. The herb should not be used by pregnant or breastfeeding women, or by people who have high blood pressure, liver disease, or heart disease.

Because goldenseal is so popular, some manufacturers substitute other herbs, including Chinese goldthread and Oregon grape, which do not contain the same active components and may increase the risk of adverse events. To avoid getting an ineffective product, always purchase goldenseal supplements form a reputable manufacturer.

GREEN TEA

When was the last time you enjoyed a cup of green tea? Hopefully it was recently, as green tea *(Camellia sinesis)* has healing properties that can be helpful for people of all ages. It has been a part of Chinese and Ayurvedic medicine for thousands of years, where it has been used to improve heart health, boost energy levels, aid digestion, and heal wounds. Today's scientists are finding many uses for this plant.

Of the three main types of tea—black, oolong, and green—green tea contains the highest concentration of antioxidants called polyphenols, which are the source of the tea's healing properties. The reason for this higher antioxidant level is that green tea, unlike the other two forms, is not fermented, and so it retains more of its free-radical fighting powers than the other teas.

What Are the Benefits?

Studies show that the main polyphenol in green tea, epigallocatechin gallate (EGCG) and other polyphenols have anticancer and anti-inflammatory properties, as well as the ability to lower cholesterol. In one study, for example, green tea significantly reduced total cholesterol and "bad" LDL cholesterol in patients who took the extract for eight weeks.

In the association between green tea and breast cancer, researchers have found evidence that the polyphenols in green tea have abilities to fight breast cancer, that drinking green tea may delay the onset of breast cancer, and that green tea extracts can enhance the cancer-fighting abilities of the cancer drug paclitaxel.

How Much Should I Take?

Green tea is a remedy you can enjoy with your meals! A suggested adult dose is 2 to 4 cups of green tea daily, aiming for a total of 240 to 480 mg polyphenols. If you choose a green tea extract supplement, look for brands that provide a high percentage of polyphenols per dose, preferably 70 percent or higher. A recommended dose of standardized green tea extract in capsules is 300 to 400 mg daily. Children who weigh 50 pounds can enjoy one-third of any adult dose, while those who weigh 100 pounds can take two-thirds the dose.

Cautionary Tales

Green tea in small amounts is not believed to pose a risk to pregnant women. According to complementary medicine physician and author Andrew Weil, MD, 200 mg of caffeine daily from green tea or other beverages does not increase a woman's risk of miscarriage. The EGCG in green tea can reduce the body's ability to use folate, however, so pregnant women may want to limit their consumption of green tea to one to two cups daily, since folate is critical in preventing birth defects.

HAWTHORN

Hawthorn *(Cragaegus oxycantha)* has had a reputation since ancient times as being an herb that helps the heart, and that reputation continues today. There are several dozen species of hawthorn, but the one most often used for herbal remedies is *Crataegus oxycantha*. Traditionally the berries were used for herbal remedies, but today supplement manufacturers most often use the leaves and flowers to make their products, because they are believed to contain more active ingredients than the berries.

Those active ingredients in hawthorn are antioxidants, including quercetin and oligomeric procyandins (also known as OPCs), which destroy cell-damaging free radicals. It is believed that these antioxidants are the substances that give hawthorn its healing abilities.

What Are the Benefits?

The antioxidants in hawthorn may dilate blood vessels, protect the blood vessels from damage, and improve blood circulation, all of which make the herb helpful in lowering blood pressure and cholesterol levels. It also can be used to reduce symptoms of coronary artery disease. Do not expect to see dramatic changes overnight, however. You will need to take hawthorn daily for several months before you enjoy its benefits.

How Much Should I Take?

You can buy hawthorn supplements as capsules, tablets, liquid extracts, and crushed leaves or fruits to make infusions. Shop for extracts standardized for total flavonoid content (usually 2 to 3 percent) or procyanidins (18 to 20 percent). Dosages of hawthorn range from 80 to 300 mg of capsules or tablets taken two to three times daily, or 4 to 5 mL of tincture taken three times daily. If you prefer the tea (infusion), add 2 teaspoons of crushed leaves or fruits to 8 ounces of boiling water. Steep for 20 minutes and drink two cups daily. Hawthorn is not recommended for children.

Cautionary Tales

Side effects are rare, but may include nausea, headache, and palpitations. If you have a heart condition, you should talk to your doctor before taking hawthorn. Hawthorn may increase the effects of cardiac glycoside drugs (e.g., digoxin), cholesterol-lowering drugs, and drugs to treat high blood pressure. Do not take hawthorn if you are pregnant or breastfeeding.

LICORICE

This perennial herb is a native of southern Europe and western and central Asia. Licorice *(Glycyrrhiza glabra)* has a long tradition of use for both its sweetness and its healing properties. In traditional Chinese medicine, licorice was used to treat sore throats and food poisoning, and the ancient Greeks used it to ease coughs. Native Americans had similar uses for the roots, but also took the herb to treat diarrhea, stomachaches, and fever.

What Are the Benefits?

The licorice root contains glycyrrhizin, which is the source of both its sweet flavor and its anti-inflammatory and soothing properties. A licorice-infused cream or lotion, when applied to skin disorders such as eczema, can be just as effective as the steroid hydrocortisone in reducing inflammation and itching. Glycyrrhizin also promotes the secretion of mucous and soothes irritation. Flavonoids, other active ingredients in licorice, help heal digestive tract cells and thus make this herb helpful in treating constipation and heartburn. The flavonoids also act as antioxidants and work to protect the liver.

How Much Should I Take?

Licorice comes in two forms: standard and deglycyrrhizinated licorice (DGL). The DGL form is preferred for oral supplements because it does not cause the stomach problems associated with the standard form. However, the standard licorice (which contains glycyrrhizin) can be used safely in topical forms. For treating constipation and heartburn, 0.4 to 1.6 grams of DGL extract is suggested, three times daily. For strep throat, make a tea using about 4 grams of chopped or freshly grated licorice root added to 8 ounces of boiling water. Steep for 10 to 15 minutes and strain.

Cautionary Tales

High doses of licorice may cause serious side effects, including hypertension, heart irregularities, fatigue, and edema, so do not take more than recommended. Do not use licorice if you have diabetes, high blood pressure, or kidney, heart, or liver disease. Pregnant and breastfeeding women should not take licorice. Licorice may increase the effects of anticoagulant drugs and herbal remedies.

PEPPERMINT

Here is an herb that is a favorite for kids of all ages. Peppermint *(Mentha x piperita)* is a cross between spearmint and water mint, and an herb that has been used since ancient times for medicinal purposes and for flavoring. The plant has essential oils, and both the leaves and the oils contain menthol, which provides pain-relieving, soothing properties.

What Are the Benefits?

The menthol in peppermint's oils and leaves has the ability to relieve spasms, especially in the digestive tract. This makes peppermint a good candidate to treat colic in infants. By relaxing the muscles of the esophageal sphincter at the top of the stomach, peppermint can help release air that is trapped, thus reducing belching and bloating. Menthol can also stimulate receptors in the nostrils and can serve as a decongestant and expectorant. That's why you may find menthol/peppermint as an ingredient in chest rubs. Several studies have shown that peppermint is effective in treating diarrhea, bloating, and gas.

How Much Should I Take?

Peppermint is available as dried leaves from which you can make tea; as a tincture containing 10 percent peppermint oil and 1 percent peppermint leaf extract; as enteric-coated capsules, which are specially coated to allow the capsules to pass through the stomach and into the intestines; or as a cream (containing 1 to 16 percent menthol).

To prepare the tea, steep 1 teaspoon dried peppermint leaves in 8 ounces boiling water for 10 minutes. Strain and cool. Drink four to five times daily between meals. When treating infants who have colic, cooled peppermint tea can be given one teaspoon at a time, four to five times daily. One to two enteric-coated capsules can be taken two to three times daily. Children who weigh 50 pounds may take one-third the adult dose; those weighing 100 pounds may take two-thirds of the dose.

Cautionary Tales

Do not take peppermint if you have gastroesophageal reflux disease (GERD) or hiatal hernia. Because peppermint relaxes the sphincter between the stomach and the esophagus, the herb can make symptoms of indigestion and heartburn worse. Pregnant and breastfeeding women should not use peppermint. Do not take enteric-coated peppermint capsules at the same time you take drugs that reduce the amount of stomach acid, because the capsules may dissolve in the stomach rather than the intestinal tract.

PSYLLIUM

Psyllium is a high-fiber substance that is derived from the husks of the seeds of the *Plantago ovate,* a plant that grows in India, parts of Asia, the Mediterranean, and North Africa. The plant offers two healing substances: a very high level of soluble fiber and seeds that are coated with mucilage, a substance that is not water soluble and is not digested by the body. These two properties are the main source of psyllium's healing abilities.

What Are the Benefits?

Many studies have shown that psyllium can reduce total cholesterol and low-density lipoprotein (LDL, or "bad" cholesterol) levels after several weeks of treatment. This is one reason why psyllium is sometimes referred to as a "heart-healthy" supplement. Psyllium is also an effective treatment if you suffer with constipation and want a natural laxative, or if you need a bulking agent to treat diarrhea. Psyllium is able to work in both situations because in cases of constipation, the psyllium combines with water, swells, and produces more bulk, which stimulates the intestines to contract and helps move stool through the tract. This feature also makes psyllium helpful in treating hemorrhoids.

If you have diarrhea, the mucilage absorbs water from the intestines and makes their contents more solid. The psyllium also slows down the digestive process, which allows more water to be reabsorbed, which in turn controls loose stools.

How Much Should I Take?

Adults generally begin with ½ teaspoon of psyllium seed added to 8 ounces of warm water. Stir it well, because it can thicken quickly, which can make it difficult to drink comfortably. Gradually increase the dose up to 2 teaspoons daily as needed and depending on the condition you are treating. If you choose a commercial product that contains psyllium, follow the instructions on the package. Do no skimp on the water, as psyllium requires an adequate amount of water to work properly. Children ages six to 12 can take half the adult dose, beginning with ¼ teaspoon of psyllium seed or husks. Good news: psyllium is safe for pregnant and breast-feeding women.

Cautionary Tales

Psyllium supplements may delay or reduce your ability to absorb certain medications. To help avoid this, take psyllium at least 1 hour before or 2 to 4 hours after taking other medications. Psyllium should always be taken with at least 8 ounces of water, and you should drink at least 6 to 8 glasses of water throughout the day to avoid constipation. Do not take psyllium if you have difficulty swallowing or you have any narrowing or obstruction of the gastrointestinal tract. Some people who take psyllium experience some gas and bloating, which is a potential side effect from any fiber product.

PYCNOGENOL

Pycnogenol® is the trade name of a natural plant extract derived from the bark of the French maritime pine tree *(Pinus pinaster* spp. *Atlantica)* that grows in France. The bark contains various substances that are known to have healing qualities, including proanthocyanidins (OPCs), bioflavonoids (including catechins), and organic acids.

The constituents in the pine tree extract are credited with several basic properties, including antioxidant, anti-inflammatory, and aiding in the production of nitric oxide, which helps to dilate blood vessels.

What Are the Benefits?

A recent (January 2010) study found that both oral and topical pycnogenol resulted in significant improvement in people who had hemorrhoids. Symptom relief was faster in patients who used both oral and topical pycnogenol, but the herb was effective in patients who were treated with only one form as well. Hemorrhoidal bleeding was eliminated in all the patients who were treated with pycnogenol for seven days.

Pycnogenol has also been beneficial for reducing hyperactivity and improving concentration and attention in children who have ADHD. It appears that the herb reduces stress hormone levels, which in turn improves symptoms of ADHD. For people who have diabetes, pycnogenol may lower glucose levels and also be helpful in treating retinopathy, a common complication of diabetes in which the blood vessels in the eye leak.

How Much Should I Take?

Pycnogenol is available in tablets and capsules. In the studies of pycnogenol and ADHD, the children were given 1 mg of the herb for every kilogram (2.2 pounds) of body weight on a daily basis. Before giving your child pycnogenol, talk to your doctor. For treating diabetes, the suggested dose for adults is 100 to 200 mg daily in divided doses. For treatment of hemorrhoids, the oral dose ranges from 150 to 300 mg daily. The topical cream is available in 0.5 percent potency and can be applied several times a day to the affected areas.

Cautionary Tales

Although preliminary research indicates that pycnogenol may be safe for women in late pregnancy, it is best to not use this herb if you are pregnant or breastfeeding. Pycnogenol rarely causes side effects when taken as directed. Some people have experienced dizziness, headache, stomach distress, and mouth ulcers. Because pycnogenol might increase the activity of the immune system, it could worsen symptoms of autoimmune diseases such as lupus, rheumatoid arthritis, and multiple sclerosis. Therefore it is best to avoid pycnogenol if you have an autoimmune condition.

QUERCETIN

Quercetin is a plant pigment found in the barks and rinds of a wide variety of plants. In the diet, it is found in large amounts in apple skins, onions, tea, and red wine, and in lesser amounts in berries and leafy green vegetables.

What Are the Benefits?

Quercetin is a potent antioxidant that helps protect the body from free-radical damage to the cells, which contributes to aging, heart disease, cancer, and other diseases. In respiratory conditions such as asthma, allergies, hay fever, and sinusitis, quercetin inhibits the production and release of histamine and other chemicals that cause inflammation and allergy symptoms.

Several studies have shown quercetin to be effective in relieving symptoms of chronic prostatitis (swelling of the prostate gland). Quercetin also works with other bioflavonoids and nutrients and helps them function more effectively. For example, quercetin increases the activity and effectiveness of vitamin C. There is also some evidence that quercetin may relieve the inflammation associated with arthritis and thus reduce symptoms. Quercetin is also sometimes promoted to help prevent or treat cancer.

How Much Should I Take?

A suggested dose of quercetin is 50 to 200 mg three times daily for adults. Quercetin supplements should not be used by children less than one year of age. Older children may take it at a dose that is one-quarter to one-half an adult dose, beginning at the low end for youngest children. Quercetin is available in tablets and capsules. Makers of a special type of quercetin, called quercetin chalcone, say it is absorbed better, but there is little evidence to prove this claim.

Cautionary Tales

Quercetin appears to be safe. Although it "failed" a standard lab test called the Ames test, which helps identify chemicals that may be cancer-causing, most other evidence indicates that quercetin may actually help prevent cancer. Maximum safe dosages for young children, nursing women, and people who have serious kidney or liver disease have not been established.

SLIPPERY ELM

Slippery elm *(Ulmus fulva)* was a favorite herb among Native Americans for use in healing salves for wounds, burns, and skin inflammation, and orally to relieve sore throats, coughs, diarrhea, and stomach disorders. The tradition lives on, and today slippery elm is used for some of the same purposes.

The remedy comes from the slippery elm tree, which is native to North America. The inner bark is dried and powdered to be used in herbal supplements.

What Are the Benefits?

Slippery elm contains mucilage, a substance that can coat and soothe the throat, mouth, stomach, and intestinal tract. The herb also has antioxidants that can help relieve inflammatory bowel disorders, diarrhea, and ulcers. In a study conducted at Queen Mary's School of Medicine and Dentistry, for example, slippery elm demonstrated its antioxidant properties and promise as an effective treatment for inflammatory bowel disease.

How Much Should I Take?

Slippery elm is available in tablets, capsules, lozenges, powdered bark for making tea, and coarsely powdered bark for poultices. Children's doses are one-third to two-thirds the adult dose, depending on the child's weight. Suggested dosages for adults include 400 to 500 mg three to four times daily taken with a full glass of water; 5 mL three times daily of the tincture; and three cups daily of tea, prepared by pouring 16 ounces of boiling water over 2 tablespoons of powdered bark and allowing it to steep for 3 to 5 minutes. Lozenges should be used according to package instructions.

Cautionary Tales

Slippery elm is not associated with any serious side effects. Because the herb coats the digestive tract, it can reduce the absorption of other drugs or herbs. Therefore, take slippery elm two hours before or after you have taken medications or other herbs. Although slippery elm is believed to be safe, pregnant or breastfeeding women should not take it.

ST. JOHN'S WORT

Ancient people believed that St. John's wort *(Hypericum perforatum)* could drive out evil spirits and help treat nervous disorders, but today the shrubby plant has assumed some different purposes, although not completely! St. John's wort is one of the most commonly purchased herbal products in the United States, and among the many ailments it is used for is mood disorders.

St. John's wort contains many components, but researchers have focused on hypericin and pseudohypercin, which are believed to be the active ingredients. These substances are found in the flowers and leaves, which are used to make supplements.

What Are the Benefits?

Today, the main use for St. John's wort is treatment of depression. Extensive research shows that St. John's wort can reduce depressive symptoms in people who suffer with mild to moderate depression and can be just as effective as both tricyclic antidepressants and selective serotonin reuptake inhibitors, but with fewer side effects. It may also be helpful in relieving mood swings associated with PMS. The herb is also used for several other conditions, including skin conditions such as eczema and minor burns.

How Much Should I Take?

St. John's wort is available in capsules, tablets, tinctures, teas, and oil-based lotions. Look for supplements that are standardized to contain 0.3 percent hypericin. If you choose to take tablets or capsules, the typical dose ranges from 300 to 500 mg three times daily. The liquid extract can be taken at a dose of 40 to 60 drops twice daily. Take St. John's wort with meals. If you want to make an infusion, add 1 to 2 teaspoons of dried herb to 8 ounces of boiling water and steep for 10 minutes. Drink up to two cups daily. It can take up to eight weeks before you enjoy the benefits of St. John's wort.

For treating skin conditions such as eczema, look for a 1.5 percent hyperforin cream, which can be applied to the affected area as directed on the package, typically twice a day.

Cautionary Tales

Potential side effects are usually mild and may include dry mouth, dizziness, headache, fatigue, rash, or stomach distress. If you use the cream, use sunscreen while you are being treated with the herb, because St. John's wort may cause the skin to become overly sensitive to sunlight. Do not use this herb if you are pregnant or breastfeeding.

STINGING NETTLE

Stinging nettle *(Urtica dioica)* is an unpopular weed but a welcome healing remedy for a variety of symptoms and ailments. Since ancient times, stinging nettle has been used for conditions ranging from arthritis to anemia and skin disorders. Both the leaves and stems, and sometimes the roots, of the plant are used for healing purposes. The roots have different healing properties than the leaves and stems.

The fine hairs on the leaves and stems of sting nettle contain irritating chemicals that are released when the plant makes contact with the skin. Although these spins are normally painful to the touch, they actually decrease pain when they make contact with a painful part of the body. Scientists believe nettle has the ability to reduce the levels of inflammatory chemicals in the body and thus interfere with the way the body transmit pain messages.

What Are the Benefits?

The most common uses for stinging nettle today include hay fever and allergies, as research shows that the herb helps reduce sneezing and itching. This ability is believed to be due to nettle's ability to reduce the amount of histamine the body produces in response to an allergen. Stinging nettle leaves and stems are also used to treat bronchitis and asthma, while the roots are used for treatment of an enlarged prostate (benign prostatic hypertrophy). The herb is often an ingredient in creams used to treat joint pain, sprains, and insect bites.

How Much Should I Take?

Stinging nettle is available as dried leaves, extract, capsules and as a root tincture. Adult doses can be reduced by one-third for children weighing 50 pounds or two-thirds for those weighing 100 pounds. To prepare a tea, add 6 ounces of boiling water to 3 to 4 teaspoons of dried leaves or dried root and steep for 3 to 5 minutes. Drink 3 to 4 cups daily. For capsules containing dried leaves, take 2 to 4 grams three times a day. For the fluid extract of the leaves, take 2 to 5 mL three times daily.

Cautionary Tales

Stinging nettle is generally considered safe when used as directed. Occasional side effects may include fluid retention, mild stomach upset, and rash. If you use the topical form, do not apply to an open wound. Because nettle can alter the menstrual cycle, pregnant women should not use this herb.

Stinging nettle may interfere with the body's ability to clot blood and with blood-thinning drugs, such as warfarin and clopidogrel. The herb may lower blood pressure, which means it could affect any blood pressure drugs you are taking. It may also act as a diuretic, and could increase the risk of dehydration if you are taking other diuretics.

TEA TREE OIL

Tea tree oil is an essential oil that is obtained by steam distillation from the leaves of the *Melaleuca alternifolia* plant, which is a native of Australia. At one time the leaves were used as a substitute for tea, which is how this tea tree oil got its name. Today, however, it is the oil that is valued for its healing purposes. Among the constituents in tea tree oil are terpenoids, which have antifungal and antiseptic properties. One terpenoid in particular—terpinen-4-ol—is the most abundant and believed to be the one that has the most antimicrobial abilities.

What Are the Benefits?

People use tea tree oil to treat acne, athlete's foot, dandruff, vaginitis, gum problems, and skin disorders, and there are studies to back up many of these uses. One study looked at the use of 25 percent and 50 percent tea tree oil solution or placebo in people with athlete's foot. After applying the tea tree oil twice daily for four weeks, 64 percent of the people who used the 50 percent tea tree oil were cured, compared to 31 percent in the placebo group. Another study found 100 percent tea tree oil to be just as effective as clotrimazole, an antifungal medication, in treating fungal infections of the toenails.

In acne studies, 5 percent tea tree oil significantly reduced inflamed and non-inflamed acne lesions and was associated with far fewer side effects than benzoyl peroxide, the usual medication used to treat acne.

How Much Should I Use?

Tea tree oil is available as a pure essential oil, and it is also an ingredient in creams, lotions, and ointments. For treating acne, diluted tea tree oil can be applied with a cotton swab to the affected areas several times a day and allowed to stay on overnight. Wash off the oil in the morning. Because tea tree oil is potent, dilute it with aloe gel. Add one to two drops of tea tree oil per ounce of aloe gel. If this combination does not irritate your skin, you can gradually increase the amount of tea tree oil that you add to the aloe. You can also use a commercial tea tree oil lotion.

Cautionary Tales

Some people are sensitive to tea tree oil and experience itching, redness, or irritation. These reactions are most likely to occur if you use undiluted tea tree oil, but can be avoided or significantly reduced once diluted with aloe gel, vitamin E oil, or even olive oil. Tea tree oil should not be used internally. Pregnant and breastfeeding women should not use topical tea tree oil.

VALERIAN

Valerian is an herb that is native to Europe and Asia, but now it is grown around the world. The root is believed to house the active ingredients of the herb—valerenic acid and bornyl—in its essential oil. The one that supplements are often standardized to is valerenic acid. Like most prescription tranquilizers, valerian appears to have an impact on a neurotransmitter called GABA in the central nervous system.

What Are the Benefits?

The most common use of valerian root is as a sedative, to help people sleep and to treat anxiety. Valerian remains popular in the United States and Europe even though many doctors now write orders for prescription drugs to treat these disorders. Studies of valerian in adults with sleep disturbances have found that the herb improves the quality of sleep and reduces the amount of time it takes to fall asleep (sleep latency) for up to four to six weeks.

How Much Should I Take?

Adults typically take 150 to 300 mg extract standardized to contain 0.8 percent valerenic acid, or ¼ to ½ teaspoon (103 mL) valerian tincture several times daily. Valerian is also often used as a tea, with 1.5 to 3 grams of the root steeped for 5 to 10 minutes in 6 ounces of boiling water.

Cautionary Tales

If you take the recommended amounts, the risk of side effects is very low. Occasionally valerian can cause stomach upset, while at large doses it can cause headache, nausea, grogginess in the morning, and restlessness. Pregnant and breastfeeding women should not take valerian. Do not take valerian for longer than two months, as it can actually cause insomnia at that point. If you have been using high doses of valerian for several months, you may experience withdrawal symptoms (e.g., rapid heartbeat, confusion) if you stop taking it suddenly.

GLOSSARY

Antioxidants: Substances that prevent damage to cells from molecules known as free radicals or from oxidation. The body produces its own antioxidants, but it also needs supplies from the diet. Some dietary antioxidants include vitamins C and E, beta-carotene, selenium, copper, zinc, and phytonutrients.

Bioflavonoids: Compounds found in fruits that contain vitamin C. You will sometimes see bioflavonoids listed on vitamin C supplements.

Chelated: This term refers to minerals that are attached to proteins, which increases their bioavailability. Look for chelated minerals when shopping for minerals.

Coenzyme: A nonprotein molecule that attaches itself to a protein molecule to form an active enzyme that can participate in chemical processes.

Daily Value: A term that replaces the RDA (Recommended Dietary Allowance) on food labels. It refers to the percentage of the recommended daily amount of a substance that each serving or supplement dose provides.

Dietary Reference Intakes (DRIs): A category of values

that are the standards for nutrient intake for healthy individuals. The values are based on the average requirements for different sex and age groups and include Recommended Dietary Allowance (RDA), Tolerable Upper Intake Level (UL), Adequate Intake (AI), and Estimated Average Requirement (EAR) values.

Fat-Soluble Vitamin: A vitamin that can be dissolved in fat and is stored in fatty tissue in the body. Fat-soluble vitamins include vitamins A, D, E, and K.

Flavonoids: Also known as bioflavonoids, they include any of a large category of phytonutrients that are plant pigments.

Free Radicals: Unstable molecules that attach themselves to other molecules, cause damage to the cells, and can result in disease and other health problems.

Neurotransmitters: Chemicals produced by the brain and nerves that transmit and change nerve signals.

Phytoestrogens: Plant chemicals that have a structure similar to the hormone estrogen but have only a very mild estrogenic effect.

Phytonutrients: Nutrients that are derived from plants, especially ones that are neither a vitamin nor mineral.

Polyphenols: Potent antioxidants that belong to a class of phytonutrients. The word means "many phenols," with a phenol being a type of carbon-based molecule.

Water-soluble Vitamins: Vitamins that the body does not store, and so you must replace them daily through diet and supplements. The B vitamins and vitamin C are water-soluble.

APPENDIX

HERBAL INFORMATION

Alternative Medicine Foundation, Inc.
PO Box 60016
Potomac, MD 20859
www.amfoundation.org/herbinfo.htm
Comprehensive information on herbal remedies

American Botanical Council
6200 Manor Road
Austin, TX 78723
www.herbalgram.org
Comprehensive information on herbs

American Herbalist Guild
141 Nob Hill Road
Cheshire, CT 06410
www.americanherbalistsguild.com
Nonprofit educational organization; can help you find an
    herbalist

HerbMed
An interactive, electronic herbal database that provides in-
    formation courtesy of the nonprofit Alternative Medicine
    Foundation
www.herbmed.org

GENERAL HEALTH AND NUTRITIONAL SUPPLEMENT INFORMATION

American Dietetic Association
www.eatright.org
Lots of nutritional information and help finding a registered
  dietitian

Association of Accredited Naturopathic Medical Colleges
4435 Wisconsin Avenue NW, Suite 403
Washington, DC 20016
www.aanmc.org

Center for Food Safety and Applied Nutrition
www.cfsan.fda.gov/~dms/supplmnt.html
Government website with the latest on food safety and nutritional information

Center for Science in the Public Interest
www.cspinet.org
Advocates for nutrition and health, food safety, school food,
  etc.

Consumer Lab
www.consumerlab.com
Provides independent information and test results on nutritional products

Dietary Supplement Information Bureau
www.supplementinfo.org
Provides information on the responsible use of nutrients,
  herbs, and specialty supplements

Dietary Supplements Labels Database
http://dietarysupplements.nlm.nih.gov/dietary
Information about the ingredients in more than 4,000 dietary
  supplements sold in the United States

Food and Nutrition Information Center
http://fnic.nal.usda.gov/nal_display/index.php?info_
    center=4&tax_level=1

Health A to Z
www.healthatoz.com
Comprehensive information on consumer health topics

Health Central
www.healthcentral.com
Comprehensive information on consumer health topics

Linus Pauling Institute
http://lpi.oregonstate.edu
Comprehensive information and research on nutrients

Mayo Clinic
http://www.mayoclinic.com
Comprehensive overviews on a wide range of consumer
    health topics

National Center for Complementary and Alternative Medi-
    cine
http://nccam.nih.gov

National Institutes of Health
www.nih.gov

Nutritional Tree
www.nutritionaltree.com/default.aspx
Publishes consumers' reviews of nutritional products. No ad-
    vertising is accepted on this website

U.S. Department of Agriculture, My Pyramid
www.mypyramid.gov
Offers personalized eating plans and interactive tools to
    make informed decisions about nutrition

U.S. Pharmacopeia
www.usp.org
An independent public health organization that provides information on dietary supplements

Wrong Diagnosis
http://www.wrongdiagnosis.com
Provides information on symptoms, diagnosis, and misdiagnosis of more than 10,000 medical conditions